The Healing Field

M.T. Morter, Jr., B.S., M.A., D.C.

The Healing Field,

by M.T. Morter, Jr., B.S., M.A., D.C.

ISBN# 0-944994-03-2

Printed in Rogers, Arkansas

© 1991, Best Research, Inc.
1000 West Poplar
Rogers, Arkansas 72756

The Healing Field

Table Of Contents

Introduction 1

Chapter 1
Healing's Rites of Passage 5
   External Forces and Health 6
   Medicine Turns Inward 10

Chapter 2
The Abstract Materializes 15
   Viewing the Vital Body as a Machine 18

Chapter 3
Fields: The Unseen Cradle of Health 23
   Fields of Health 24
   External Electromagnetic Fields 26
   Effects of Electromagnetic Fields
   on the Human Body 27

Chapter 4
What Others Say About Electromagnetic Fields 31

Chapter 5
Harnessing Energy of Electromagnetic Fields 37
   Electromagnetic Currents of the Body 39
   Internal Space 40

Chapter 6
What Others Say About Frequencies of Energy 43

Chapter 7
Our Link With the Past 49
   Fields of Development 49
   Embryogenesis 51
   Developmental Information 52
   Cellular Communication 56

Chapter 8
    What Others Say About Information and Communication ... 59

Chapter 9
    Communication Through Fields 73
        A View of the Unseen Fields 75
        Electron Information 77
        Fields of Information 78
        Unlimited Interrelationships 80
        Communicating Change 81

Chapter 10
    What Others Say About the Influence of Fields and Currents 83

Chapter 11
    Rhythmic Patterns of Life 93
        Physiological Pulsations 94
        Anatomical Pulsations 96
        Tapping into the Universal Pulses 99

Chapter 12
    What Others Say About Physiologic Pulses 101

Chapter 13
    Reconnecting the Mind 109
        Surviving to Defend While Defending to Survive 111
        Self Esteem and Self Disdain 113
        Mind, Thoughts, and the Universal Energy 114
        Dynamic, Vibrating Energy 116

Chapter 14
    Intentional Healing 119
        Resonating With Health 119
        Tuning the Field 121
        Content and Intent 123
        Negative Intent 124
        Intent, Double Blind Studies, and the Placebo Effect 127

Chapter 15
    Working with the Healing Fields 131

References
    Books 137
    Journals and Periodicals 141

Introduction

*"Once the idea has been grasped in essence, then
the details may be examined afterwards."*
— Penrose p. 428

Bio Energetic Synchronization Technique (B.E.S.T.) began to evolve in 1972 in response to clinical observations of patients' responses to adjustive procedures. "Inventing" or "devising" another chiropractic technique was not my aim. My purpose as a chiropractor was to help sick people get well. In my previous five years of practice, I had been extremely successful in terms of patient volume, and at least conventionally successful in patient improvement. However, the morning I observed, in ten consecutive patients, that adjusting one area of the spine affected another area of the spine marked the beginning of change in my professional focus, and, I believe, will ultimately mark the beginning of the expansion of the focus of chiropractic and health care.

B.E.S.T. has evolved in response to the needs of patients. The procedures have been, and continue to be, demonstrated as clinically effective. *Clinical effectiveness in both relieving pain and enhancing health is the primary goal of B.E.S.T. When health is present, pain and disease are unnecessary.*

In the process of developing procedures that enhance health to relieve pain, I did not search scientific literature for clues as to what might work. On the contrary, I found procedures that worked, and used them. In time, I realized that any procedure that is consistently effective must be based on scientific truths. Years later, I began to investigate literature. In my search for truth, I have found evidence of many research projects and scientifically accepted concepts that confirm my clinical findings and explain why B.E.S.T. procedures are effective. Quotations from some of these references are interspersed where appropriate in the text, and presented in bulk in the sections "What Others Say. . . ." The quotations in these sections are in chronological order to give the reader a flavor of the progress of thought toward "energy medicine." We can see by the writings of others that B.E.S.T. concepts are not "new." The development of B.E.S.T. procedures has been parallel with findings and concepts detailed by others, yet has not been tied to verification by outside sources.

Direct quotations from a variety of authors appear in the "What Others Say..." sections. These quotations are indented for ease of identification. Comments not indented are mine. All italics that appear in direct quotations are those of the author quoted and are shown as they appeared in the source cited.

I believe that advancements in technology will confirm, for those professionals truly intent upon improving the health of mankind — those in both research and clinical practice — the ultimate influence on health and disease of energy: electrical, gravitational, magnetic, and their concomitant fields.

Scientific researchers are uncovering more and more evidence of the importance of electromagnetic fields in our lives. Excessive exposure to man-made fields created by electrical and electronic equipment is currently receiving a great deal of attention as a contributor to a variety of ailments and diseases from headaches, brought on by long-term exposure to energy from computers, to cancer, attributed to living in close proximity to high-voltage equipment. Information and research findings are pointing toward energy fields playing a greater part in the function of the body and health than had previously been considered.

In our mechanistically-oriented society and culture, effects, such as symptoms, are attributed only to those causes that can be quantified and treated by therapies, chemicals, or surgery. Yet we will see by the evidence presented in the following pages that electromagnetism can be a greater influence on physiology than is currently "accepted."

The human body develops from the union of one egg and one sperm forming a single cell. From this one cell grows a complete individual who ultimately is made up of trillions of cells. Each of these cells contains information identical to that in every other cell in that body. The level of information is not divided as the cells divide. Where does the information come from in the first place? What intelligence prompts one cell to differentiate to function as a part of an eye while another cell, containing the same information, differentiates to function as a part of a tibia? In addition, what prompts the organized growth of any living system? How does a developing embryo know to form a child or fish?

Researchers suspect that information is contained in cells. Holographic evidence reveals the outline of a completely formed system around the seed of that system. Evidence supports the concept that information is contained in the fields around living systems. The healer's role, then, is to help the patient affect his or her fields in order to bring the body back into harmony and synchrony with these fields in order to allow fluid communication of the information between the fields. When interference in the transmission of information from field to body is removed, the body is able to conform itself to the ideal configuration of the field.

A dominant hypothesis of B.E.S.T. is that the body (diseased or healthy) is a reflection of the field, and the field is a reflection of the energy radiated by the body.

The principal energy generator of the body is mental activity: cortical and subcortical. Thoughts and attitudes emit energy. Negative thoughts and attitudes reduce and interfere with the energy of the controlling field. Conversely, positive thoughts and attitudes project positive energy to the field and allow positive energy to be received from the field. Even more startling, negative or positive energy projected by the doctor's thoughts and attitudes (intent) in the presence of a patient can markedly affect the patient's physical response. We can extrapolate from this concept to understand the placebo effect. If the doctor and/or patient believes that the "medicine" will be effective, the belief is generally realized. Intent can be more powerful than content.

Bio Energetic Synchronization Technique procedures, in conjunction with the patient's and doctor's attitudes, bring about positive results for most patients. The explanation of exactly why B.E.S.T. helps patients improve has been long in coming and continues to be explored. Yet, by applying the concepts of energy fields — electrical, gravitational, and magnetic — to health, a greater understanding of pain and disease is possible. Approaching patients' complaints from this perspective explains the many instances of inexplicable diseases and discomforts. Now, the doctor can understand why some patients chase from doctor to doctor, clinic to clinic, and end up with a verdict of "We can't find anything wrong."

The reason "nothing can be found" in many patients who suffer severe afflictions is that only the physical and chemical aspects of the body are being considered. The body is greater than the sum of its parts — much greater. And the body is the only source of its own health. Doctors can't heal; medicines can't heal; surgery can't heal; and, worst of all, chiropractic adjustments can't heal. The body heals itself. Any and all externally administered treatments address effects only, and the effects are responses of the body striving to survive. Every function of the body is perfect for the conditions under which it is functioning. Pain and disease are effects of the body functioning in the best manner to survive. The way the body is functioning — either in harmony with its environments in a healthy state, or in disharmony with its environments in a disease state — is necessary. In order to successfully help patients improve, the *need* for disease must be eliminated.

— M.T. Morter, Jr., B.S., M.A., D.C.

". . . we must work with nature rather than trying to improve on it."
— Robert O. Becker, M.D.

1

Healing's Rites Of Passage

*One of the greatest pains to human
nature is the pain of a new idea.*
— Walter Bagehot, 1826-1877

The road to our present state of medicine and healing has been rocky, filled with detours, and marked with potholes of contention. The roles of assorted cultures have been equally as important as that of man's intellect in this journey. Throughout history, thoughts that run counter to the prevailing norm — scientific or philosophical — have met with scorn, derision, punishment, or death. Jesus of Nazareth, Copernicus, and Martin Luther King are but a few of the men who have altered the course of man's thinking with ideas that disrupted established beliefs.

The course of the development of the philosophy and practice of medicine has not been a smooth, continuous upward climb to our present level, nor will the future course be uncluttered by dissention. Medicine and healing deal with intangibles just as surely as they deal with tangibles. History has shown that man's attitude toward the source of health and disease has taken what might appear to be a cyclical journey from a holistic view to a mechanistic view and, now, is running back again to a holistic view.

As technology has advanced over the centuries, man has been able to investigate farther reaches of outer space and smaller components of nature and the body. With each enlargement of our known cosmic universe and each reduction of our elemental structures comes additional knowledge that sometimes decimates long-held cultural or "scientific" beliefs. In addition to stacking discovery upon discovery, science is a progression of exchanging one view of the microscopic or cosmic worlds for another. For example, Harvey's discovery that the blood circulates in a closed system opened the door to understanding the operation of countless processes in the body, and modern space exploration has revealed previously unknown electrical activity in space.

We build our cultural and independent beliefs on the information available to us. One of the premises of this book is that all information is available; our reception of it is limited only by our knowledge.

External Forces And Health

For our early ancestors, body, mind, spirit, circumstances, and health were inextricably interwoven. The two realities of life — the physical world that could be seen and the spirit world that was unseen — determined present and future health and fortune. Spirits had to be appeased, placated, and "bribed." Circumstances, both personal and corporate, were determined by forces unseen yet absolute. Since recorded history, man has attributed "spirit properties" to all living things. Lives were at the mercy of the whims of an invisible vital "life force," or energy.

From the times of the shaman and the witch doctor, man has attempted to explain his circumstances, life, and health in terms of a governing entity: gods and/or the forces of nature either smiled upon or punished man for his actions — intentional or not. Illness was treated by offerings or supplications to a variety of deities or other power brokers. Strong, invisible forces were believed to control man and his environment. Health or disease was externally dictated by nature and the gods, and treatments were solicited from nature and the gods.

Imhotep, the Egyptian architect-priest-magician-physician of the third century B.C. who was seen as a demigod a scant hundred years after his death, believed "that unseen forces live in the elements." According to this chief magician/physician of pharaoh's court, "evil spirits" (unseen forces) were responsible for many physical ills. (Bach, p.25) No physical evidence disputed this belief, and a great deal of circumstantial evidence confirmed it; people became sick for no apparent reason. Logic indicated, the sufferer must have done something to attract the attention of evil spirits.

Evidence from as early as 2000 B.C. shows that the Chinese recognized the lifeforce of *Chi* and its energy concepts of *yin* and *yang*. These principles continue to be recognized and ministrations based on these principles are still used — apparently quite successfully — by Eastern practitioners.

However, Western medicine had its beginnings with Hippocrates about 500 B.C. Perhaps best known by the general public for the Hippocratic Oath that outlines a code of conduct for physicians, Hippocrates taught a philosophical approach to medicine, cited diet as a major factor in disease, and viewed disease within the framework of the patient's lifestyle.

Hippocrates apparently taught at the medical school on the Greek island of Cos where he was born in 460 B.C. Medicine and philosophy were meshed in teachings of the Coan school; treatment centered not only on the patient and his ills, but on his entire life and surroundings. In this same era, the philosophy taught at Cnidus, situated on the opposite peninsula from Cos, focused on disease. The Cnidian philosophy took a reductionist bent to determine exact diagnoses. The forerunner of modern medicine that deals with disease specificity, the Cnidian concepts died due to lack of information and knowledge about internal organs. Cnidian medicine was born prematurely and succumbed to inadequate resources: in this instance, limitations of knowledge.

For Hippocrates, philosophy and observation were the primary diagnostic tools. His followers altered the course of medicine by rejecting the concept of supernatural forces as the sole cause of human distress. Some six hundred years later, the Greek physician Galen introduced scientific experimentation to provide greater opportunities for observation.

Through his analysis, anatomical dissections and inspections of the wounds of gladiators, Galen contributed a vast amount of knowledge concerning the "form and function" of the internal organs and structure of the human body. Galen was perhaps the first "researcher" to define the location, purpose, and function of specific organs while he perpetuated the long-held belief that disease was brought about by an imbalance among the four "humors": blood, yellow bile of the liver, black bile of the spleen, and phlegm of the brain.

As elementary as the concept may seem to us now, it was Galen who first determined that the diaphragm and thoracic muscles expand and contract the chest cavity to fill the lungs rather than the lungs filling to expand the cavity. Galen was so convinced, and convincing, that he had uncovered the secrets of the human body, further study was considered unnecessary. Explanations of functions he had not observed were provided through his philosophical theses that were accepted as equally valid as the verifiable. Interpretations (and sometimes mis-interpretations) of Galen's writings were the basis not only of European teachings but of Moslem and Arabic-speaking Jewish teachings as well.

Galen's teachings were so thoroughly accepted that the course of "scientific" investigation was stifled. Rather than students learning from their own investigations of anatomy, they were regaled with readings from Galen by their physician-professor while a barber-surgeon dissected a cadaver. Galen's observations and writings were considered so comprehensive that for nearly fifteen hundred years medical progress was at a standstill.

Paraclesus, German-born physician, alchemist, and teacher, was one of the first to rail against the stifling teachings of Galen, and he rejected "the prevailing view that the stars and planets controlled all the parts of the human body." (Britannica, 9:134) His early exposure to theories of chemistry and metallurgy in the early 1500s led him to the realization that "miners disease" (silicosis) was brought about by "inhaling metal vapors and was not a punishment for sin administered by mountain spirits," and that "carefully measured doses of mercury compounds taken internally" could successfully treat syphilis. Through his proclivity for chemistry, he laid the foundation for the practice of homeopathy declaring that, in small doses, "what makes a man ill also cures him." (Britannica, 9:135) Paraclesus was a transition figure from the dogmatic Galenic teaching to a combination of modern-day chemical therapy and the concept of the power of natural healing. "A Paraclesian axiom was that everything in the universe is related to every other thing and that, 'Everything God made is good for something, it is merely a matter of relating the goodness' " (Bach, p. 145). The bombastic Paraclesus did not accept Galen's iron-clad dogma, even going so far as to burn his books as an act of defiance. His radical ideas and his practice of opening his lectures and knowledge to the general public rather than restricting them to students incensed the authorities of his day.

Yet, the second-hand method of teaching and learning medicine and surgery of Galenic principles continued until 1543 A.D., the same year Copernicus received the first printed copy of his book that showed the sun rather than the earth to be the center of our solar system. This was the year that twenty-eight-year-old Andreas Vesalius published *De Humani Corporis Fabrica*. "Anatomy begins with this book, and so does modern scientific medicine," writes Nuland. It "epitomizes the confluence of science, technology, and culture in a way that few, perhaps no, other books have ever done," (Nuland, p. 62) and can be seen as opening the door to modern investigative medicine.

In 1605, although medicine was focusing more and more on specific organs, and although he investigated internal parts, Francis Bacon continued to work under the premise that disease was based on "humoral imbalance." He saw "innate heat" as the "force that acted both to maintain equilibrium and to restore it when it was lost."

John Locke (1632-1704), English physician and philosopher, resisted the "correlation between symptoms and their organs of origin." He prophesied: "Though we cut into the inside, we see but the outside of things and make but new superficies to stare at. . . . Nature performs all her operations in the body by parts so minute and insensible that I think nobody will ever hope or pretend even by the assistance of glasses or other inventions to come to a sight of them." (Nuland, p. 155)

Locke was referring to the single-lens microscope that came into use in the mid-15th century. Surprisingly, cells weren't observed until the 17th century. By 1674, however, lenses had been developed that were powerful enough for Antoine van Leeuwenhoek to observe tiny bacteria.

Locke was more correct in his prediction that man won't be able to see all of the operations of the body than would appear at first glance; we are discovering increasingly smaller components of the body and other matter, yet we still haven't isolated the "living" factor.

The emergence of scientific investigative procedures was a major step in setting the stage for succeeding greats in the history of healing. The scientific world began its move from vitalism to mechanism. Gone was the underlying premise that supernatural or ethereal elements were the basis for disease. The foundation was laid for discoveries such as Harvey's recognition of the circulatory system in the sixteenth century, and, in the early eighteenth century, Morgagni's method of observing, formulating a hypothesis, experimenting, and recording data. Morgagni provided the pattern for the clinicopathological conference, or CPC, used in medical schools today. His *De Sedibus et Causis Morborum per Anatomen Indagatis* (referred to by its shortened title *De Sedibus*) sets out case histories, autopsy findings, and observations in the form of letters that served to advance the cause of pathological anatomy.

Giovanni Morgagni championed the mechanistic approach that has come to dominate scientific thinking. He disparaged the traditional concept that imbalance of the four humors was the origin of disease and cited, instead, dysfunction of specific organs. Medicine embarked on the "anatomical concept of disease."

Medicine Turns Inward

The world of medicine was moving from the stance that the body expresses organic or systemic symptoms because it is sick, to the concept that the patient is sick because of disease or malfunction of specific entities within the body. Yet, despite the monumental progress made in understanding the intricacies of the human body, down to and including the workings of cells and DNA, we still have not come to identify the power that promotes health — or disease.

The eighteenth century saw surgeons delve more and more into the internal mysteries of the human body. Scottish-born John Hunter (1728-1793) although small of stature, was a giant among researchers. Despite his rustic personality and lack (as well as disdain) of formal education, he transformed surgery from a mechanical procedure to an experimental science. Hunter, a naturalist who reaped his education from constant observations of nature, recognized "that the answers to his questions could not be found in books." (Nuland, p. 174) Rene Laennec (1781-1826), on the other hand, was well-schooled and captured every opportunity to advance his education. It was Laennec who catapulted medical diagnosis into the age of technology with his invention of the stethoscope.

The well-known stethoscope didn't come into being through weeks or hours of intense research and development; it is the product of one man's discretion. The anecdote attached to its development may have been embellished to make the story more interesting, but medical folklore recounts the events leading up to the advent of the stethoscope. While examining an unusually voluptuous and attractive young woman who was suffering from a chest disorder, Laennec found that, due to her generously endowed configuration, palpation was ineffective and that, due to her youth and comeliness, discretion and custom precluded his employing the customary ear-to-chest procedure. Being a musician and recalling childhood games of listening at one end of a stick to scratchings at the other, he rolled up a quire of paper, placed it against the young woman's chest and was surprised and delighted with the clarity of sound he heard. Thus, the birth of the stethoscope. This invention in 1819 "was surely the Hippocratic method of observation brought forward into modern times." (Nuland, p. 221) Now, clues to internal functions could be gained by first-hand observation rather than merely through a recitation of symptoms by the patient. Although this new diagnostic tool was readily accepted as a boon to improved observation, like most deviations from the norm, it was not received without at least token resistance. Some doctors considered the instrument an affectation to impress patients. Others claimed it was either too long or too short. And, others expressed concern that patients wouldn't like it. However, detractors of the new tool soon fell into line with the majority and not only adopted its clinical use but ultimately its symbolic use as a badge of the profession.

Since the advent of the stethoscope, medical researchers have looked for clues separate and apart from the patient's description of his problem. The mid-1880s "was the period of history ... when the central point of medical research shifted from the patient to his disease," (Nuland, p. 231), as the long evolution of the microscope allowed scientists to gain a clearer picture of cells. The reductionist Cnidian philosophy was again gaining momentum.

At about the same time the stethoscope was gaining acceptance, Rudolph Virchow (1821-1902) was born in Prussia. Virchow identified the cell as the "focus of disease." Yet he championed the thesis that "a man is the product of his life situation." Virchow's views were an amalgamation of the Cnidian and Coan philosophies. The German pathologist discovered that the cell is the basis of disease, health, and life itself, and established a foundation for modern medical research. Although he followed the trend of looking at the body in smaller and smaller increments, he did not lose sight of the forest while examining the trees; he attributed the onset of the typhus epidemic in 1848 (the same year as the Communist Manifesto) to peasants being kept in a "state of moral degradation, personal filth, and indolence."

The mid-1800s brought a flurry of advances in medicine. Surgical anesthesia erupted on the scene in 1846 at Massachusetts General Hospital in Boston. This boon to mankind, the first major contribution of American medicine, has removed much of the agony of surgical and dental procedures for millions. It was perhaps the only "advancement" that met with no opposition, although, strangely enough, those to whom the development of this pain-saver is credited have been termed "enterprising mechanics, but certainly not scientists." (Nuland, p. 265) Nitrous oxide, or laughing gas, might be seen as an early recreational drug. It entered the medical arena by the back door. One of its original uses was as an entertainment device by enterprising entrepreneurial traveling "professors" that temporarily transformed deep, resonant voices into cartoon-character squeaks.

Exactly who should be given credit for discovering or inventing anesthesia has been a subject for debate. Several originators claimed the distinction for themselves at about the same time. This coincidence of time and achievement is not uncommon in developing new products or procedures. As we shall see later, information is all around us, yet until we have the resources to recognize and understand it, it goes unnoticed. Information is universal, waiting for the right receiver to observe, capture, and assimilate it.

The history of healing has followed a bumpy course of trial and error, observation and application, and dogged investigation interspersed with flashes of brilliance. Medicine has concentrated on repairing symptoms of afflictions brought about by external violence or internal abuse. The history of healing is in reality an ongoing saga of man's attempts to relieve physical distress. Hippocrates' Coan philosophy focused on observing the person as a whole — the physical being as an integral part of his surroundings and universe. The Cnidian philosophy initiated the attitude that the diseased part is the problem. We might term these deductive healing and inductive medicine: deductive healing approaching health as a function of the whole — the whole person and the universe; and inductive medicine approaching disease beginning with the most microscopic element currently known.

2

The Abstract Materializes

Man's perspective of life, the body, health, and the controlling elements of all nature has altered dramatically since his early days on earth. At the beginning, man was aware of himself and his body. He didn't know what made the body work. He knew only that he (his body) existed and was his centrality. Strength and agility were the primary means of survival, and survival was the primary goal. Stronger creatures and elements of nature were credited with powers far beyond those of man to control his life and destiny.

As civilization progressed, man determined that "humors" inside the body determined health and temperament. A predominance of phlegm resulted in a phlegmatic temperament. A predominance of bile resulted in an irascible temperament, and so on.

As time went on, western man began to learn, through the openings of wounds, the configuration of the inner body — organs, muscles, bones. And when dissection became legal and the internal structures were examined more closely, man came to understand that there was communication within the body through the nervous system, and this communication was directed by the brain.

Physicians concentrated on physical, viewable, extractable, quantifiable material objects.

Then, for those who pursued such interests, thought moved to a more abstract area that was evident but not visible — the mind. Although the mind couldn't (and can't) be singled out as a physical entity, its presence had become obvious. Man is a thinking creature. The brain could be examined, but thought processes and the results of these processes could not be excised and put into a test tube. The mind, whatever it is, is

THE HEALING FIELD

abstract. Evidence indicated that the mind has a definite effect on the body despite the fact that the mind couldn't be extracted and examined under a microscope.

Now, the abstract mind is beginning to be credited with more influence on the physical body than had previously been accepted. However, it still can't be quantified. And, some scientists are going even further than that. They are climbing to the next level of abstraction in health investigations. Evidence now points to energy fields as influencers of both the mind and the body.

Perhaps, after we have accepted the mind's influence completely, we will learn even more about the energy fields and realize that they are an even greater influence on health than the mind. When we have accepted the concept of mind-influence wholeheartedly, we will begin to learn more about the fields which, in turn, will begin to open up the next level of abstraction. As more is learned about the relationship among energy fields, the mind, the body, and health, perhaps evidence will point to yet another level of abstraction as the ultimate controlling power.

Forward thinking men appear to think a step-and-a-half beyond where "conventional wisdom" is comfortable. While the conservative majority continues to function at the "accepted" level of thinking and beliefs, forward thinkers move to the next level of abstraction.

Who knows where it will end — probably not at the energy fields. Until science has reduced the human body and other living systems to such minute intervals that they will find nothing left — space — scientific investigations will continue to focus on purely physical, chemical, and biological reactions to explain and try to mend the body's ills.

Twentieth-century science has made giant strides in isolating and identifying ever smaller components of matter: both external matter credited with causing disease, and internal components that bring about the symptoms of disease. Yet, science still has not identified or quantified the invisible ingredient that constitutes the "living quality." Nor has science succeeded in identifying, locating, or quantifying the "mind." Despite these omissions of verification, the concept of the mind is fully accepted, and the relationship between mind and body

The Abstract Materializes

has been the subject of discussions, arguments, and writings by learned men for centuries. The 17th century philosopher/mathematician, Rene Descartes, coined the oft-quoted philosophical maxim: "I think, therefore I am." It was Descartes who, undaunted by lack of an answer to how mind and body interact, formulated the concept of dualism, or separateness, of mind and body. In the second half of the 1880s, Sigmund Freud, scientist and the father of psychoanalysis, searched for physiological and materialistic explanations for his theories of the psyche.

Throughout the history of healing, two threads are interwoven: the Coan philosophy that when the person is ill, the whole person is ill, and the Cnidian philosophy that illness is confined to specific locations, segments, or organs.

With this background, D.D. Palmer and chiropractic walked boldly onto the healing stage. In 1895, D.D. laid the foundation for the procedures that came to be termed "chiropractic" — an amalgamation of the Coan and Cnidian concepts of deductive healing and inductive medicine.

D.D. Palmer stressed the age-old premise that everything in the universe is controlled by a universal intelligence which is the fundamental health-seeking property of the body. He termed this intelligence "Innate." Both D.D. Palmer, discoverer and developer of chiropractic, and his son after him, B.J. Palmer, promoter and "missionary" of chiropractic, saw Innate as "intuitive, instinctive, and immortal" (Bach, p. 102). D.D. set the tone for future chiropractors and patients by insisting that two types of intelligence exist within each of us — educated intelligence that we glean through the personal experience of years of living, and Innate intelligence with which each of us is born.

Palmer's methods of healing (then as now) met with remarkable, often seemingly miraculous, results. Chiropractic proponents and patients grew in numbers as word of this non-invasive form of therapy spread. However, chiropractic has stumbled along paths similar to those trod by medicine in that progress has been less than smooth. Resistance to the structure-function model by established healing disciplines has been strong, taking forms ranging from slurs and innuendoes by laity speaking from a position of ignorance, to

THE HEALING FIELD

vehement disavowal of concepts, philosophy, and procedures by the AMA speaking from an adversarial position. Dissention has also erupted within the ranks of chiropractic, pitting those who espouse the use of hands-on-spine only to others who have sought to incorporate additional therapeutic elements.

Much of the contention appears to revolve around the mechanistic vs. vitalistic philosophies.

Viewing The Vital Body As A Machine

As civilization moved out of the Dark Ages, scientifically learned men laid the groundwork for an attitudinal shift from that of viewing man as controlled by natural or supernatural forces to man the mechanic — the fixer of things gone wrong. Scrutiny of ever smaller components of the body revealed how the body works. Anatomy and experimentation were beginning to reach a state of art. In the early seventeenth century, Francis Bacon, although he considered disease to be based on "humoral imbalance," wrote, "We must question what we can't see and test our ideas with experiments." Search for the cause of illness was moving from the corporate universe to individual anatomical structures and physiological processes.

The early Greeks had seen the source of illness as a combination of an individual's basic nature, environment, and external stimuli. As knowledge progressed, Morgagni identified sick organs as the origin of disease, Bichat cited sick tissue within as the culprit, and in the late-nineteenth century, Virchow credited the cell as the "basic unit of disease...health, and of life itself." (Nuland, p. 307) Yet, Virchow perpetuated the "thesis that man is the product of his life situation." (Nuland, p. 315) Virchow's viewpoint was an amalgamation of both Hippocrates Coan school of thought and the Cnidian approach, and heralded the shift to the physician focusing on the patient's disease rather than on the patient himself. Treatment revolved around altering the course of physiological chemical reactions. However, medicine had not yet become rigidly controlled to concentrate exclusively on drug and surgical therapy or to exclude innovative concepts.

Around the turn of the nineteenth century, the German M.D. Samuel Hahnemann, picked upon reports that when quinine was administered to healthy patients, they expressed symptoms of the disorder quinine was used to cure. From this observation, Hahnemann formulated his theory that "likes are cured by likes," based on the "law of similars." From this observation grew the healing discipline of homeopathy. Although with homeopathic treatment, drugs are usually administered in minute doses as opposed to the large, system-shocking doses of modern medicine, critics of homeopathy cite that even these procedures focus on the disease they are trying to cure rather than on finding the cause of the disease.

Man has taken for himself the role of "fixer" or "mechanic." He has assigned the body the role of machine, the working parts of which must be tuned, adjusted, repaired, replaced, and kept in running condition by the intelligence of the mechanics. The tools used to fix the machine are predominantly drugs and surgery. As scientific knowledge concerning the chemical aspects of cellular function has increased, medicine has flourished using the chemical model. We, as a society, now view disease predominantly as a chemical malfunction of organs, tissue, and cells. Since a considerable amount is now known about how healthy systems, organs, tissue, and cells function, and with this knowledge modern technology can usually pinpoint where the problem lies, most of today's disease-fighters put their confidence and expertise in trying to adjust chemical reactions in the body. Disease and other disorders are considered specific: they are seen as "abnormal" conditions affecting only circumscribed components of the body. Too often, the mechanistic approach looses sight of the patient as a whole and only sees "a cancer," or "diabetes," or "osteoporosis," or the latest disease-to-end-all-diseases, "AIDS." A disease or illness takes on a persona of its own, defined by diagnostic tests and calculations, reinforced by prognostications, and singled out for attack. The disease itself is treated as an entity separate and distinct from the individual patient. Only cursory attention is paid to lifestyle (overeating, drinking alcoholic beverages, smoking, lack of exercise), and even less attention to the patient's external environment, attitudes or thought patterns. *We, as a scientific community and as a people, are "too sophisticated" to believe that intangibles such as thoughts and energy and fields of the universe impact our lives or our health.*

The mechanistic approach operates on the premise that the smarter we get about how microscopic elements of the body work, the more we are able to control disease. In reality, however, no matter how smart we get, no matter how much we know about the way the body works, we'll never be able to scientifically document "life" or creation. We'll learn about the *effects,* but we'll not be able to explain just what life is or pinpoint the moment of creation. As with our concept of electricity, we cannot define the life force. We know how it works and how to use it, but we don't have any idea of what it is — We can see the effects of electricity, but we can't see electricity itself. Similarly, we'll never be able to see "life."

The scientific revolution that led to the establishment and refinement of mechanistic medicine has fed man's senses and provided the basis for the edification of medicine. Scientific knowledge is predominantly a cortical function. It stresses verification, replication, and logic. This is a laudable stance. Yet it limits man's advancement in the healing arts to his current knowledge.

The mechanistic approach limits advancement in the art of healing and health to the parameters defined by our conscious knowledge. The mechanistic approach functions under the premise that the body is simply a machine that cannot heal itself and that the only effective therapies are powerful drugs, surgical invasion, and mechanical technologies. (The mechanical approach and technology have been exploited to the point that medicine is rapidly pricing itself out of a job.)

The mechanistic approach is satisfying and comfortable for many doctors, both medical and chiropractic. It confines their diagnoses and therapies to visible, verifiable, measurable, quantifiable, specific areas of the body. Yet patients are more than a mere conglomeration of physical parts. The many parts of the body function as a unit. A more highly sophisticated intelligence and communication network keeps the diverse organs and systems functioning in perfect tune with each other. Disharmony among the individual parts, or congestion or interference in the communications network result in what we term symptoms. Many of the functions of the body are controlled by segments of the brain that transmit orders, without conscious thought, to secrete or stop secreting fluids or hormones, increase or decrease blood pressure, alert the

The Abstract Materializes

immune system, or perform all of the other physiological functions of which the patient is unaware.

Along with the internal world of activity over which they have little control, patients live in a world of seen and unseen forces: gravitational, electrical, magnetic, even cosmic.

Our forefathers credited natural and supernatural forces with the power to bestow life, or induce or cure illness. They were aware that a form of energy influenced their persons and their environment. When these forces were favorable, life existed. When they were lacking, life ceased. For lack of a better definition, they attributed these forces to gods and spirits and "humours." These forces are the same now as they were then; the difference is that we have attached names to them, such as electricity, gravity, and magnetism, and are becoming increasingly aware of their nature and ubiquity. We now know that these forces are forms of energy and that all matter —including the human body — is energy. We are moving rapidly into the era that recognizes the impact of energy on health and even life itself.

Energy produces fields around itself and around concentrations of matter. Everything is a form of energy. Not only are matter and man energy itself, this energy is constantly in motion, colliding, and forming new fields. Each new field that comes about from the combination of two or more fields is a form of creation. We are constantly in a stage of creation. Every thought we have "creates" a new energy field to blend with the other fields around it. The idea that "thoughts are things" is not an original concept with me. More and more "mechanists" as well as "vitalists" are beginning to understand that the energy of thoughts determines whether the body runs synchronously in health, or dis-synchronously in disease.

Despite our space-age-years' revelations of electrical and electromagnetic energy throughout our universe, the application of this knowledge has not been pursued by main-line medicine. Have we, at the end of the twentieth century, fallen into the same trap as those of the early seventeenth century of believing that we know all there is to know? Like the followers of Galen who believed that knowledge of the human body was complete, we have acknowledged that chemicals alone drive the body and there is no need to look to another source of vitality. However, as our scientific technology improves, some of our observations disagree with accepted dogma of healing. These observations force expansion or change in our concepts of healing.

The purpose of this book is to share with other doctors and seekers-after-truth my observations and conclusions of over twenty-five years of investigation into the cause of disease and health. I will focus on natural healing and how our internal and external environments mandate either disease or health. For the mechanistically minded, I shall incorporate findings from scientific research that underscore the conclusions formed from clinical observations that led to the development of the Bio Energetic Synchronization Technique (B.E.S.T.).

B.E.S.T. might be viewed by some as a naive reversion to pre-renaissance thinking that the body is governed by "humours" and "spirits," and that when these nebulous, invisible entities are out of sorts, the body becomes sick. On the contrary. The B.E.S.T. philosophy recognizes the monumental strides made by modern and pre-modern scientific thinkers and researchers such as Harvey and Morgagni in determining how the body functions, and that disease strikes at specific organs and areas of the body. B.E.S.T. philosophy re-introduces the dimension of holism, not to refute learned concepts but to use them in conjunction with the theory that reductionism has not yet gone far enough to get to the seat of health.

Indeed, disease is manifest in specific organs and tissues, and these diseases can be treated — sometimes successfully, sometimes unsuccessfully. B.E.S.T. philosophy posits that specific malfunctioning organs and tissues are not the origin of the problem — they are result of systemic upheaval. B.E.S.T. is a systemic approach to health, and the whole body is a system — visible, palpable, measurable, and physical — working within other systems.

3

The Unseen Cradle Of Health

The purpose of this chapter is to lay a foundation for the principles and procedures of the application of Bio Energetic Synchronization Technique. The procedures focus on finding and eliminating the primary cause of neurological interference as opposed to concentrating on restructuring symptoms. Subluxated vertebrae are symptoms of interference, just as blood flowing from a lacerated foot is a symptom of a wound. Stanching the flow of blood from an open wound is desired. Obviously, unrestrained loss of blood can be fatal. However, bleeding is not the problem; the wound is the problem. Bleeding is a sign that a problem exists and is an effect of the problem. Subluxations, like bleeding, diabetes, cancer, multiple sclerosis, and all other collections of symptoms are not the cause of ill health; they are indicators.

Symptoms indicate interference in the transmission of information, or knowledge, that directs the body's functions. Interference is caused by timing, toxicity, or thoughts. Of these, thoughts are the most potent interference-producers. Timing and toxicity are results or effects; they are end-products of the body responding to stimuli. Timing and toxicity can be seen as passive or reactive. They are the result of conditions imposed on the body. Timing and toxicity can be evaluated through clinical or laboratory examinations. They are quantifiable, and they can be altered by external stimuli. Timing is altered through adjustments. Toxicity is altered by changing lifestyle or diet. Timing and toxicity are conditions defined by man's conscious mind. Patients may or may not know that their timing is off or that their bodies are toxic.

Thoughts, on the other hand, are energy. Thoughts can't be captured on film, seen under a microscope, or excised with a scalpel. Thoughts themselves cannot be quantified, yet the effects negative thoughts have on the body can. Negative thoughts transmit negative energy that disrupts the electromagnetic fields in and around the body. How this occurs will be discussed at length in other sections of this book. First, a look at the source of electromagnetic fields that are influenced by thoughts and that play a major role in health.

Fields Of Health

Scientific research has shown that there is little question that electromagnetic fields not only exist but that they influence living systems. The question of degree of influence on human health will be widely debated in the 21st century as public pressure demands a return to a holistic view of the body that allows for a more effective and complete form of health care. From the B.E.S.T. perspective, electromagnetic fields not only exist but, as will be discussed, are seen to be the means of communicating with extra-conscious aspects of the physical body: the subconscious and superconscious faculties of the brain and mind.

The human body is a more complete entity than casual observation would suggest. Around every living system (including each patient) is an energy field that is electromagnetic in nature and an integral part of that system. Not only does each entity, such as a patient, possess its own electromagnetic field, but each component of that entity, cells, tissues, and organs, and the atoms and electrons that make up those components, is encapsulated in its own field. Contiguous fields blend to influence one another, thereby creating yet another field. Because electrons, protons, atoms, molecules, and all other apparently distinct structures are constantly moving and coming in contact with other structures, the field of one contacts and interacts with field of another. Consequently, the electromagnetic fields of any living being are constantly in a state of change. Each field influences and is influenced by other fields with which they come in contact, thereby creating yet another field. The human body, therefore, might be described as a teeming mass of electromagnetic activity.

Since the fields and the physical body of the patient influence one another, complete healing can take place only when both the field and body are in a state of equilibrium. Maximum healing is possible only under conditions of complementary physiological homeostasis and field homeostasis, i.e., the fields of the body are in tune with, or resonate harmoniously with, the fields of the universe.

B.E.S.T. philosophy postulates that disease and physiological distress are both causes and results of disruption of the fields surrounding the body. This premise, although not yet "scientifically accepted," is also espoused by other advocates and students of the vitalistic principle and all-encompassing holistic healing. Gabriel Cousens, M.D., in his introduction to Gerber's *Vibrational Medicine*, espouses the view of the holistic principle and the question of holistic balance. Dr. Cousens states that ". . . we, as human organisms, are a series of interacting multidimensional subtle-energy systems, and that if these energy systems become imbalanced there may be resulting pathological symptoms which manifest on the physical/emotional/mental/spiritual planes." (Gabriel Cousens, M.D., author of *Spiritual Nutrition and the Rainbow Diet*, Gerber, p. 28)

Electromagnetic fields serve both as the energy to fuel the functions of life and the pattern to shape life.

Gerber cites Burr's research of electrical fields surrounding seedling sprouts that showed the shape of the field surrounding the seedling resembled the mature plant rather than the sprout itself; and Burr's data suggest "that any developing organism was destined to follow a prescribed growth template and that such a template was generated by the organism's individual electromagnetic field." (Gerber, p. 52)

Becker terms electric and magnetic fields "abstractions" that help scientists to understand phenomena that are "undeniable" but have no readily identifiable source. "Physicists have been trying for generations to solve the fundamental mysteries of electromagnetism, and no one, not even Einstein, has yet succeeded." (Becker and Selden, p. 81)

Although exactly what electromagnetism is and exactly where it comes from is still a scientific mystery, the existence of electromagnetic fields in and around the earth and other matter cannot be denied. Furthermore, studies have shown that these unseen fields can affect health. B.E.S.T. takes this concept a step further: not only do the fields exist and have an impact on health, *fields are the vital communication link between man and the universe*, and the information communicated among these fields ("nous" in theological circles) is a primary determinant of health. This is a major hypothesis of B.E.S.T. philosophy.

External Electromagnetic Fields

The concept of fields around the earth and around matter that moves with the earth is well established. "Around every particle, whether it be at rest or in motion, whether it be charged or uncharged, there are potential fields of various kinds." (Britannica, 26:494) Electric and magnetic fields exist around electric charges. Electric fields are brought about by the interaction of opposite electrical charges, i,e., positive and negative. Magnetic fields that change in intensity are associated with moving electric charges. (Britannica, 26:494)

Magnetic fields are part of everyday life. In addition to the earth's built-in electromagnetic fields, man-made high-tech and low-tech equipment contribute additional fields that produce changes in our environmental magnetic fields. Homes, offices, factories, and laboratories all contain electrical equipment that produce exposure levels of various degrees. Electric shavers, drills, toasters, microwave ovens, and the multitude of other electrical appliances common to households in the western world impose various magnetic flux densities on their immediate and close-range surroundings. "While for some time it has been tacitly assumed that electric fields are more effective than magnetic fields in interacting with biological systems, many recent studies indicate the importance of magnetic fields as well." (Stuchly, p. 215)

Investigation into the impact magnetic fields have on human biological systems is in its infancy although the question has tantalized man since Scottish physicist James Clerk Maxwell proposed his electromagnetic theory in 1864. However, interest in the sphere of influence of magnetic fields on physiological reactions has taken something of a back seat to interest in electrical fields. "Magnetism," Becker states, "is a dimly understood intrinsic property of matter that manifests itself in two polarities." (Becker and Selden, p. 81)

We are exposed continuously to electromagnetic fields. Even without the electrical fields generated by modern technology, we are and have always lived enveloped by electromagnetism. Just as marine creatures exist in their fluid medium (of which they are probably oblivious), so too we live bathed in electromagnetic forces (equally oblivious to the medium).

The electromagnetic field of the earth itself measures about 0.5 gauss, and, although this measurement is relatively static, it varies slightly on a yearly basis. (Becker and Selden, p. 107) Man-made equipment affects our electromagnetic environment. "Prevalent exposures to time-varying fields are at the power-line frequency and are mostly due to electrical appliances and power distribution systems. ... In some industrial, scientific and medical applications exposures to much stronger, both static and time-varying, magnetic fields occur." (Stuchly, p.223)

Effects Of Electromagnetic Fields On The Human Body

Ample evidence cited in scientific papers and the popular press leaves little doubt as to the existence of electrical fields in and around living systems. Where electricity exists, magnetic fields exist: around atoms and around the earth. In 1976, with nearly twenty years of research into "Magnetism and Living Bodies," Kyoichi Nakagawa, M.D., a Japanese researcher, summarized some of his findings concerning the influence of the earth's magnetic fields on the human body. This paper reflects Nakagawa's concern that a magnetic field deficiency syndrome "for a certain human body" is manifest in "some abnormalities." Nakagawa states: "...there is a direct relationship between the decrease in the earth's magnetic field acting on the human body and the improvement of abnormal conditions of the human body by the application of magnetic fields." (Nakagawa, p. 1)

The researcher cites a variety of symptoms that can be attributed to a magnetic field deficiency: symptoms ranged from stiff muscles to chronic constipation to headaches to "general lassitude." " ... In other words," writes Nakagawa, "it is a syndrome in which no objective pathological findings can be noticed from routine physical and clinical examinations, but in which the subjective symptoms persist and are hard to improve, resisting various treatments but responding to the application of a magnetic field. An unbalanced autonomic nervous system or part of such might be included in this syndrome." (Nakagawa, p. 1)

Nakagawa's conclusion that less energy reaches the body in pathological conditions coincides with the B.E.S.T. premise that interference in energy flow is the primary cause of disease and subluxations. A dysfunctional body does not effectively use the energy available to it. B.E.S.T. assumes an adequate quantity of energy is available to the human body. This assumption conforms to Nakagawa's assertion that utilization of magnetic fields "is not an insertion of electrical energy into the body [rather] it is only a conversion of a part of the motion energy of the body fluid into electrical energy through the medium of a magnetic field." (Nakagawa, p. 6)

Electrical energy and electromagnetic fields have been shown to have an effect on physiological activity. Becker reports on a study of "several hundred subjects" conducted by Rutger Weaver to determine if or how electromagnetic fields affected "body temperature, sleep-waking cycles, and urinary excretion of sodium, potassium, and calcium." (Becker and Selden, p. 248) Elaborate measures were taken to isolate the subjects and to reduce the number of variables. Two identical rooms were constructed that shielded the subject from any indication of the passage of time. One room was shielded from electromagnetic fields; the other was not.

Subjects stayed in the rooms for as long as two months. Subjects "in both rooms soon developed irregular rhythms, but those in the completely shielded room had significantly longer ones." (Becker and Selden, p. 248) Subjects in the semi-shielded room developed rhythm aberrations but eventually settled into a new rhythmic pattern such as a two-day cycle rather than one-day. Those completely shielded from the earth's electromagnetic field "became thoroughly desynchronized. Several variables shifted away from the rhythms of other metabolic systems, which had already lost the circadian rhythm, and established new rates having no relationship to each other." (Becker and Selden, pp. 248-249)

When electrical and magnetic fields were gradually reintroduced, normal patterns were restored by "an infinitesimal electric field (0.025 volts per centimeter) pulsing at 10 hertz." (Becker and Selden, p. 249) Becker goes on to link the frequency of "biocycles" with the earth's electromagnetic field. "In light of this work, the fact that 10 hertz is also the dominant (alpha) frequency of the EEG in all animals becomes another significant bit of evidence that every creature is hooked up to the earth electromagnetically through its DC system." (Becker and Selden, p. 249)

These are but a few examples of research findings that solidify the connection between electromagnetic fields and physiological responses. Additional illustrations can be found more and more both in scientific publications and in the popular press.

A phenomenon witnessed by a group of doctors at the B.E.S.T. certification seminar in October 1990 provided evidence of the relationship between external fields and physiology that can have a major impact on chiropractic. The participants were intently involved in the Level III practicum required for certification. The requirement for satisfactory completion of the exercise was for each doctor to treat the patient and achieve even leg-lengths as the indicator that the patient was balanced. This exercise was being conducted in a large meeting room with over sixty doctors participating. Most of the doctors experienced little difficulty in illustrating their proficiency. However, despite the efforts of a small group of doctors in one corner of the room, their "patients" wouldn't balance. Since each of the doctors was a successful, experienced B.E.S.T. practitioner, these "failures" were perplexing. After a while, one of the doctors noticed a computer that had been used for an earlier demonstration was in that corner of the room, and it was still turned on. As soon as the computer was turned off, the doctors who had been experiencing frustrating difficulty, easily and quickly balanced their "patients."

The difficulty the doctors encountered should not have come as a surprise to any of us since the seminar material being presented focused on the impact of electromagnetic energy on the human body. This incident illustrated a common human failing: we sometimes neglect to apply our knowledge and beliefs in situations other than the customarily defined settings, such as the office.

4

What Others Say About . . . Electromagnetic Fields

With time and experience, I have come to realize that the electromagnetic fields surrounding every living system are the focal point of health. Health can be described as the body (or any other living system) functioning in symmetry and balance with its visible and invisible environment. Electromagnetic fields can be measured; yet, electromagnetic fields cannot be seen. Only the effects of fields are directly observable as readings of highly sophisticated, delicate instruments. It is by observing the effects that we understand the presence of fields. In the same vein, it is only through observing effects that we have reached our present limited understanding of health.

Potential gradients and polar differences exist in living systems. Since this is so, then electro-dynamic fields are also present.

The following theory may then be formulated. The pattern or organization of any biological system is established by a complex electro-dynamic field which is in part determined by its atomic physio-chemical components and which in part determines the behavior and orientation of those components. This field is electrical in the physical sense and by its properties relates the entities of the biological system in a characteristic pattern and is itself, in part, a result of the existence of those entities. It determines and is determined by the components.

More than establishing pattern, it must maintain pattern in the midst of geophysical flux. Therefore, it must regulate and control living things. It must be the mechanism, the outcome of whose activity is wholeness, organization, and continuity. The electro-dynamic field, then, is comparable to the entelechy of Driesch, the embryonic field of Spehmann, and the biological field of Weiss .

The Electro-Dynamic Theory of Life stated above was developed with the collaboration of Dr. F.S.C. Northrup, of Yale, and was first put forward in a joint paper in 1935. [Burr, p 33. 1972]

...to try to determine by measuring a variety of systems whether there are *always* electro-metric properties in a living organism. So, over the last thirty years, almost every form of living organism has been studied, some of them quite cursorily and others in more detail, from bacteria up to and including man. *And so far as our present information goes, there is unequivocal evidence that wherever there is life, there are electrical properties.* [Burr, pp 46-47. 1972]

The evidence of Kirlian high-voltage photography suggests that diffuse superconductive plasmas are present in clouds surrounding all solid objects, and especially surrounding living systems. [Cope 1980, p 352-353]

The body is run by a bevy of electric impulses; the heartbeat, sight, hearing, movement and many other biological activities are produced by currents passing along nerves. And, where there's an electric current there's a magnetic field. [James p 74. 1980]

Humans are governed by electrical currents. So, these currents' counterparts — biomagnetic fields— are no less than a new window looking into the workings of our bodies and minds. [James p 113. 1980]

...scientists peg the earth's magnetic field at .5 gauss. ... the magnetic field of the heart is around 1 *millionth* of 1 gauss; that of the brain plummets to about 1 *billionth* of 1 gauss. [James p 74. 1980]

During the past 15 years or so, magnetic fields produced by the human body have been measured. These fields are very weak, in the range of 10^{-10} to 10^{-5} gauss (G), and are measured with the sensitive magnetic detector called the SQUID (superconducting quantum interference device). The body's fields are produced either by naturally occurring electric currents in the body or by contaminating ferromagnetic particles. The electric currents, which consist of the flow of ions, can be either fluctuating current or steady current. [Cohen, *et al.*, p 1447. 1980]

In attempting to understand the mechanism of the touch-dcMF [dc magnetic field] we have looked for its dcP [dc potential] equivalent in the literature. Although a touch-dcP has been seen and studied, it was seen in hairless areas such as under fingernails. Hence hair follicles are not involved and the phenomenon appears to be different from ours. [Cohen, *et al.*, p 1450. 1980]

Because the dcMF over the forearms was absent over the atrophied forearms of the polio victims and present over the scar of a normal forearm, its source must intimately involve the muscles, not the skin. [Cohen, *et al.*, p 1451. 1980]

The static field across the cell membrane of all living cells, as well as the involvement of field changes in nerve impulses, is well known and intensely studied. The presence of essentially sinusoidal fields in and about cells has only very recently been established. The present paper describes a particularly simple and electrodeless technique for displaying the ac field distributions about living cells. Tiny dielectric particles of two types — those seeking field maxima, or those avoiding them — are let settle freely about the cell in a hanging drop. Patterns displaying the field distributions shortly develop that are reminiscent of those formed by magnetizable particles about a magnet. [Rivera, *et al*, p 43. 1985]

. . . SQUID for short, is a magnetic field detector thousands of times more sensitive than any previously known.... The SQUID has also confirmed the existence of the direct-current perineural system, which, especially in the brain, produces steady DC magnetic fields one billionth the strength of earth's field of about one-half gauss. [Becker and Selden, p 240. 1985]

. . . scientific effort and accomplishments are lagging behind developments in other relatively young fields such as biological effects of electric fields or radiowave and microwaves. In recent years there seems to be an increased interest in biomagnetic phenomena. Medical devices employing magnetic fields are finding beneficial applications. While for some time it has been tacitly assumed that electric fields are more effective than magnetic fields in interacting with biological systems, many recent studies indicate the importance of magnetic fields as well. [Stuchly, p 215. 1986]

In the Tiller-Einstein Model of negative space/time energies (i.e., ME or magnetoelectric energy), we have an energy which operates at speeds beyond that of light velocity. Tiller's model places the etheric spectrum of energies as moving at velocities between the speed of light and 10^{10} times the speed of light. [Gerber, p 315]

The fundamentally *new* ingredient in our picture of physical reality as presented by Maxwell theory, over and above what had been the case previously, is that new *fields* must be taken seriously in their own right and cannot be regarded as mere mathematical appendages to what were the 'real' particles of Newtonian theory. Indeed, Maxwell showed that when the fields propagate as electromagnetic waves they actually carry definite amounts of *energy* with them. . . . It is now something familiar to us — though still a very striking fact — that radio waves *can* actually carry energy!" [Penrose, p 187. 1989]

. . . a nerve signal creates a detectable changing *electric* field in its surroundings (a toroidal field, with the nerve as axis , and moving along the nerve). This field could disturb the *surroundings* significantly, . . . [Penrose, p 401. 1989]

. . . there is a continuous energy exchange between the individual and the environment which every living system (whether human , animal, vegetable, or even chemical) regulates in terms of its own self-organization. . . . it can be regarded as a universal field effect. [Shafica, p 12. 1989]

It is now generally believed that all the fundamental forces of nature — gravity, the weak and strong nuclear forces, as well as electromagnetism — possess gauge symmetries, albeit of a more complicated kind, and that these forces are transmitted by the exchange of 'gauge particles.' [Davies, p 2. 1989]

Some far-sighted theorists spotted that the success of QED [quantum electrodynamics] was based on the crucial gauge symmetry, and that the weak force might possess a form of gauge symmetry too, but one which is hidden from us. . . . nature performs the trick of hiding the gauge symmetry of the weak force. This enabled [theorists] to reformulate the theory of the weak force in such a way that it could be amalgamated with the electromagnetic force to produce a consistent theory of an integrated *electroweak* force. . . . electromagnetic and weak forces were not independent, but part of a more embracing scheme. [Davies, p 2. 1989]

... energetic mechanisms have been shown to be the basis of many of the underlying control systems that regulate the complex chemical mechanisms. [Becker, p 27. 1990]

5

Harnessing The Energy Of Electromagnetic Fields

Medical applications of magnetic fields include both diagnoses and therapies. Magnetic resonance imaging (MRI) is one of the better known, currently accepted diagnostic techniques. Magnetic fields are being used therapeutically in such areas as "field-induced hyperthermia" and a "method for magnetically removing leukemic cells from bone marrow . . . to successfully treat a child with common acute lymphocytic leukemia." (Papatheofanis, p. 252)

As investigations continue, research into healing properties of electromagnetic fields leads to various conclusions. Papatheofanis reports "that pulsed electromagnetic fields are not necessary to the induction of skeletogenesis and static intense magnetic fields may induce increased bone growth in vivo," (Papatheofanis, p. 253) Stuchly, on the other hand, reports: "Alternating magnetic fields with tailored waveforms have been used in bone fracture healing. Pulses of various shapes and repetition rates have been used . . . ." (Stuchly, p. 220) Other findings "indicate that calcified tissues are not only influenced by applied magnetic fields but that tissues themselves exhibit magnetic properties." (Papatheofanis, p. 251)

The benefits of pulsed electromagnetic field (PEMF) treatments for bone non-union are becoming more widely accepted. Treatment with pulsed electromagnetic fields is also beneficial for nerve regeneration and repair, according to a study reported by Dr. A. M. Raji of the Royal College of Surgeons of England.

Raji's closely controlled experiment using twelve pairs of male white rats revealed that significant results can be obtained through PEMF treatment. "In twelve pairs of animals, the left common peroneal nerve was sectioned and immediately sutured just above the level of the knee joint." (Raji, p. 105) All of the rats were exposed to the same pre-operative, operative, and post-operative care. Following surgery, half of the subject rats received electromagnetic pulse treatment, and half received "sham" treatments. Even the observer was unaware of which machine was the "sham."

The results of this study were significant. The treated rats began to use their affected limbs on the 12th day following the operation while untreated rats did not use their affected limbs in the same way until the 21st day following the procedure.

"At three, four and eight weeks there was histological, cytological and statistical evidence suggesting more vigorous regeneration in treated animals." (Raji, p. 111) Animals treated with PEMF following a surgical procedure fared better than those who did not.

Electromagnetic properties are now beginning to be used under controlled conditions to influence physiological functions. These natural properties have affected living creatures since time began.

The influence of geomagnetic fields on the navigation and orientation of birds, and data including a positive correlation established "between geomagnetic activity and convulsive seizures in humans strongly suggest an intimate linkage between the nervous system and applied magnetic fields." (Papatheofanis, p. 253) Additional evidence strongly suggests "a link between the pineal gland and the sympathetic and autonomic nervous systems" as contributing "to geomagnetic orientation by animals." (Papatheofanis, p. 253)

Magnetic fields of both the earth and entities on the earth influence physiology. Burr describes the results of numerous studies to confirm the existence of fields around all living systems and the association of those fields with the development and anatomical growth of that system. Burr theorized that an "electro-dynamic" field both influences and is influenced by "the entities of the biological system." (Burr, p. 33) *The electromagnetic field around each living creature not only affects the living entity, it is also affected by that entity.* The remarkable concept that the body-field influence is reciprocal bears heavily on the procedures and results of Level III applications.

Electromagnetic Currents Of The Body

The physical body as a whole can be viewed as an "effect." That is, every element of the physical body has developed in response to a stimulus of information being transferred through at least one medium. The media include chemical, electrical, and magnetic properties. Every activity of the body — hormonal secretion, enzyme activity, muscular contraction and relaxation, and nerve impulse transmission — is stimulated by one of these media. Each stimulus to which the body responds was prompted by a response to another stimulus. Most chemical reactions are instituted by stimuli of light, heat, or electricity. Muscle activity is stimulated by chemical or electrical elements. Nerve impulses are electrical charges conveyed through chemically favorable environments. It appears that the stimulus for every activity of the body involves an electrical component, and electrical activity creates electromagnetic fields. As the body functions, fields are created or changed. An electromagnetic field is stable around direct current, however, the field "collapses and reappears with its poles reversed every time the current changes direction." (Becker and Selden, p. 81) Although the intensity of both electric and magnetic fields diminish with distance from their source, the influence of the field is infinite. As fields collide and interact, they form new fields which, in turn, contact other new fields, and the process continues indefinitely. Extrapolating from this premise, we can see that when atoms collide in Cincinnati, the effects reverberate across the country, world, and outer space.

Both electrical charges and chemical reactions involve the movement of electrons. Electrons are everywhere all the time. They are not fixed entities. Electrons have been described as "the universal constituent of matter." (Britannica, 18:204 2a) Electrons have both wavelike and particulate characteristics. Electrons may move from one molecule to another to form ions. "Any flow of electrons sets up a combined electric and magnetic field around the current, which in turn affects other electrons nearby." (Becker and Selden, p. 81) The human body is a collage of force fields.

By studying a variety of species from bacteria to man over a thirty year period, Burr concluded that *"so far as our present information goes, there is unequivocal evidence that wherever there is life, there are electrical properties."* (Burr, p. 47) These properties, specifically, the electrical gradient, were demonstrated in man by using a silver-silver chloride electrode and a salt solution. Electrodes were introduced into a salt solution held in two cups. Each laboratory staff member who doubled as a subject dipped the index finger of the right hand into one cup, and the index finger of the left hand into the other cup to form a completed external circuit. The exercise was repeated and the resultant currents were measured over "many days." Rarely did a subject show a magnitude of less than two millivolts, and some were higher. Initially, all subjects were males, so female subjects were conscripted to check gender influence on the findings. The results of the measurements of voltages produced by females over time, unlike the males, showed a marked increase in the voltage during a twenty-four hour period. Investigation showed that the peak voltage readings occurred at approximately the middle of their menstrual cycles.

This development was a strong evidence of *"a change in voltage gradient associated with fundamental biological activity."* (Burr, p. 49)

Internal Space

Electrons move. Movement implies space in which movement can take place. Matter, consisting of atoms and molecules, contains undefined space. Electrons spin and orbit the nucleus in the unrestricted space of an atom. Since the body is made up of matter, we can see that the body includes unoccupied space. "Subatomic particles are separated by huge gaps, making every atom more than 99.999 percent empty space." (Chopra, p. 96)

The area in which electrons move can be viewed as space within the body but not necessary a part of the body. A broad analogy could be made with the space of the lumen of the intestine which is confined within the body but not a part of it. Areas of anatomical space are influenced by stimuli that incite activity of contiguous entities; Brunner's glands that line the walls of the duodenum, for example, affect the environment and activity of the duodenum. However, neither the lumen of the analogous intestine nor the space in which electrons move have, *as yet*, been credited as being stimulus receptors in their own right. Even so, scientific understanding of ever more minute areas of the body constantly advances, and this perception may change.

Consider the structure of cytoplasm. Prior to the development of the electron microscope, the cytoplasm of cells was understood to be a jelly-like mass that merely surrounded organelles and filled apparently unoccupied areas of cells. When ultra-high-powered instruments became available, the mass that had been thought of as nondescript was seen to contain a vast network of minute interconnecting canals of the endoplasmic reticulum.

Areas that today are considered "space" may, in the future, be found to contain substances which currently are unidentified yet which serve a distinct purpose — possibly that of intercellular communication. A hypothesis of B.E.S.T. posits that the spaces within the body in which electrons orbit and move make up the medium which harbors and transmits Innate information throughout the body.

Obviously, the information referred to here is not that which is received through the sensory system and processed by the central nervous system. Innate information, available to the body through intrabody space, is more fundamental to life than is sensory information or even genetic information. Sensory information concerns present-time conditions; genetic information concerns hereditary conditions; Innate electron information concerns universal conditions unhampered by time.

According to the B.E.S.T. hypothesis, space information continuously influences electromagnetic characteristics of the physiological system. Space information alters the physiological system which, in turn, sends altered signals back to influence the space information. It is a perpetual interchange.

Characteristics of space (outside) and system (inside) constantly influence each other, therefore constantly change each other. As information is transmitted, the receiver is changed. The receiver (the internal system) then becomes a transmitter that sends signals altered by the information back to the field (external space).

If system energy resonates synchronously with space, health ensues. If system energy is asynchronous with that of space, pain and/or disease ensues. When asynchronous communication is disrupted and man responds to his own information, he "feeds on himself. " We are "eaten up" with pain, disease, and malfunctions.

6

What Others Say About . . . Energy Frequencies

Science and the public alike accept the fact that massive amounts of energy, in whatever form, are deleterious to the function of the body: energy in the form of electricity, compression waves, sound, heat, and, even, light. Researchers are now finding evidence that supports a concept B.E.S.T. has taught for years: Extremely subtle forms of energy affect living systems.

On April 24, 1948, at Yale University School of Medicine, *hypnosis was electro-metrically recorded for the first time and compared with field shifts during other state changes.* As hypnotic states themselves involve electro-magnetic flux and reflux, Maxwell's equations can be blamed for inadvertently resurrecting that much maligned ghost, Mesmer's 'animal magnetism', now more suitably based on the laws of modern field physics. (From: Ravitz, Leonard J., M.S., M.D., F.R.S.H., "Electro-Magnetic Field Monitoring of Changing State-Function Including Hypnotic States," published in *Journal of American Society of Psychosomatic Dentistry and Medicine*, Vol. 17, No. 4, 1970.) [Burr, p 157. 1972]

The development of new techniques of very high sensitivity has now led to the experimental detection of probable superconductive transitions in organic solids (various cholates) at temperatures as high as 277°K.

The findings are of broad significance, because indirect evidence suggests that organic superconduction plays a controlling role in various functions of living systems at physiological temperatures. [Cope (1978), p 233]

Experimental evidence of superconduction in organic solids at high temperatures was obtained recently by Wolf and Halpern. These findings required the use of new instrumental methods for the measurement of extremely small changes in magnetic susceptibility and electrical resistance. Transitions (abrupt changes) in field were observed in bile cholates (4 rings with various side chains). X-ray diffraction patterns were observed to be unchanged at temperatures across the transition temperature, demonstrating that no change had occurred in the structure of the atomic lattice. Therefore the observed transitions must have been due to electronic rearrangements. [Cope (1978), p 234]

Extrapolation of the experimental data on cholates suggests that cholesterol, a major constituent of nerve and other tissues, may superconduct at physiological temperatures and above. If so, cholesterol might be a site of superconduction in living systems. [Cope (1978), p 234]

... the evidence for high temperature superconduction in organic solids raises the possibility that superconduction in solid portions of cells might play a role in living systems. Three lines of indirect evidence further suggest that biological superconduction does occur. [Cope (1978), p 235]

A role in biology for two-electron superconductive tunneling (Josephson effect) is suggested by the demonstration that numerous living systems (birds, insects, snails, and possibly man) can detect very low magnetic fields (0.5 to 1.0 G). No phenomenon other than the

Josephson effect seems to have sufficiently high magnetic sensitivity to provide the physical basis for this observed biological magneto-detection. [Cope (1978), p 235]

It's known that large amounts of this [pituitary growth] hormone in pregnancy increase the size of the cerebral cortex and the number of its nerve cells in the offspring, as compared with other parts of the brain. Ivanhoe also notes that the hippocampus and its connections with the hypothalamus are among the parts of the brain that are much larger in humans than other primates. The idea gains further support from the fact that neural activity in the hippocampus increases with electrical stimulation and reaches a maximum at 10 to 15 cycles per second, at or slightly above the dominant micropulsation frequency of today's field. The most powerful shaper of our development may turn out to be the subtlest, a force that's completely invisible to us. [Becker & Selden, p 264. 1985]

... contributions of certain individual frequencies have been identified. They are postulated to operate within normal control systems and may involve balances between synthesis and degradation. [Bassett p. 38. 1987]

This is not to say that *all* time-varying magnetic fields share the same record of safety. The energetics of other parts of the electromagnetic spectrum, for example radio frequency (R.F.), microwave and X-ray, can be harmful. Even at the lower end of this spectrum, certain frequency combinations may produce deleterious effects in some biological systems. Recent observation of possible human teratologic action of electric blankets and the impact of other types of time-varying fields on chick embryo development dictate the need for due diligence. [Bassett p. 40. 1987]

Regarding the healing of fractured bones, researchers have found that the frequency of the pulsed electromagnetic fields to which the bone is exposed is a key factor. [Gerber, p 100. 1988]

Radioactive technetium 99m was injected into the acupoints of patients, and the isotope's uptake was followed by gamma-camera imaging. De Vernejoul found that the radioactive technetium 99m migrated along classical Chinese acupuncture meridian pathways for a distance of 30 cm in four to six minutes. Injection of the isotope into random points on the skin, as well as deliberate venous and lymphatic channel injection, were unable to demonstrate similar results, suggesting that the meridians were a unique and separate morphological pathway. [Gerber, p 123. 1988]

At low frequencies of field oscillation, the energy is as Raleigh and Jeans had predicted [all energy from particles would be sucked up by the field when particle and field are in equilibrium], but at the *high* end, where they had predicted catastrophe, actual observation showed that the distribution of energy does *not* increase without limit, but instead falls off to zero as the frequencies increase. [Penrose, p 228. 1989]

Non-thermal resonant effects have also been found in the growth of yeast cultures exposed to 42 GHz microwaves. The result was a biphasic dependence on frequency, with resonance bands of 8 MHz full-width-at-half-maximum (Grundler *et al.*, Grundler,, 1985). It appears that the frequency of 8 MHz is a rather fundamental one for yeasts. [Smith & Best, p 58. 1989]

... there is a very high electric field across live biological membranes. This field is of the order of 10^7 V/m (ten million volts per meter), far greater than anything likely to be experienced by a person, even in the vicinity of overhead power lines. This field is strong enough to align all the macromolecules within a biological membrane relative to this field direction, thereby increasing their mutual interactions and their non-linear dielectric responses to eternal electromagnetic fields. Frohlich modelled this situation mathematically in terms of oscillating dielectric dipoles.... Frohlich showed that non-linear, coherent excitations of the dielectric dipoles were theoretically possible and that this could lead to long-range interactions on a very frequency-selective basis, essential if one is to have a mechanism for the selective remote control of the chemistry going on in a particular cell of the body by some distant organ which has an overseeing function for that body's activities, or to provide the organism with sensors for external fields. [Smith & Best, p 56. 1989]

7

Our Link With The Past

Fields Of Development

To fully appreciate how internal and external fields relate to health and to successful chiropractic adjustments, it is helpful to develop a clear picture of where we, as individuals, came from. It is not my intention to enter into the Creation and Evolution controversy, nor to present a treatise on sex education. However, an unbreakable link connects our understanding of health with our understanding of how the human body develops.

Much has been written about recent developments in research concerning the affect of electrical fields on physiological development of both lower and higher order embryos. Developing embryos of algae, chicks, salamanders, and frogs have shown sensitivity to electromagnetic currents. One study showed that "embryonic frog nerves, when grown in culture under the influence of an electric field, grow toward the negative pole of the field, even turning through large angles to do so. In addition, the field stimulates the growth of greater numbers of nerve projections." (Marx, p. 1149)

Evidence of electrical influence in the development of embryos is mounting. Currents emanating from an embryo are measurable outside of the embryo. Primitive beings such as algal eggs and newts have been studied to assess the presence and effects of electrical currents. Research on higher forms of life has confirmed the presence of currents during embryonic development. Researchers Jaffe and Stern report, "Recent explorations with a vibrating probe show that a wide variety of developing systems drive strong steady electrical currents through themselves. . . . substantial evidence indicates that these currents — or at least some of them — act back to affect development." (Jaffe, p. 569) The researchers measured voltage above the primitive streak of chick embryos and found that "steady currents with exit densities of the order of 100 microamperes per square centimeter leave the whole streak and return else where through the epiblast." (Jaffe, p. 569) Electrical current flows from inside the embryo to just outside the embryo then returns.

Findings of a direct electrical connection between the interior and exterior of the embryo during development supports the B.E.S.T. premise that there is a direct connection and continuous energy communication between internal and external fields.

I believe that only by accepting the major role of electrical and magnetic fields as determinants of growth and health will scientists find answers to questions such as, how do cells know what they are supposed to do? How do wounds heal? What turns off the healing process? How do arms grow to the right proportional length? Why do they stop growing?

While it is accepted that bone-length growth is governed by estrogens, understanding of the ultimate basis for cyclical production of these and other development-regulating hormones is less clear. For example, Guyton cites a phase of the female sexual cycle: "Approximately two days before ovulation, for reasons that are not completely known at present, . . . the rate of secretion of LH [luteinizing hormone] by the anterior pituitary gland increases markedly, rising six- to tenfold and peaking about 18 hours before ovulation." (Guyton, p. 971)

The hypothalamus is credited with implementing necessary physiological activity: "...secretion of most of the anterior pituitary hormones is controlled by releasing hormones formed in the hypothalamus and transported to the anterior pituitary gland by way of the hypothalamic-hypophysial portal system." (Guyton, p. 977) Guyton identifies the "mid-basal region of the hypothalamus" as being a primary influence on the rate of secretion of particular hormones. (Guyton, p. 977)

But what prompts the hypothalamus to initiate or restrict hormonal secretions? To pose the question in another way: we know that the hypothalamus regulates hormone production, however, what controls the hypothalamus? We are beginning to see that electromagnetic communication is the key.

Embryogenesis

One of the most baffling examples of structured physiological control takes place during the development of an embryo from a single fertilized egg. The zygote remains free of attachment to the endometrium until "about the seventh day following ovulation." (Guyton, p. 984) Yet during this time, the original single fertilized cell "will continue to divide in vitro as long as it is bathed in a solution of homogenized fallopian tube mucosa." (Guyton, p. 984) Researchers have established the "mechanics" of cell division and differentiation of the embryo. "Within one month after fertilization of the ovum all the different organs of the fetus have already been 'blocked out,' and during the next two to three months, most of the details of the different organs are established." (Guyton, p. 997) However, the impetus for the highly complex, interrelated processes of development is less clear. During the first week or so after fertilization, no physical connection exists between fetus and host, and for the crucial first few weeks of embryonic development, there is no central nervous system instructing the differentiation and development of the fetus.

Only after about 18 days, the ectoderm "differentiates and thickens along the future midline of the back to form the neural plate." (Noback & Demarest, p. 109) From this beginning, the brain and central nervous system are formed. The question remains: what is the source of the information that tells the cells to duplicate all of the DNA strands and to segregate them? At least two weeks elapse before there is any semblance of nervous system to control development. Yet, during this time, cells originating from one fertilized cell receive information to differentiate to form specialized cells that can perform specialized functions.

The information is not in the nervous system; early on in the developmental process, the nervous system has yet to develop. Yet the information directing development is somewhere. A cell can be totally destroyed and another one with identical abilities will take its place. The information directing a cell to multiply is outside the cell.

Cells, like all other units of matter, function within their own fields. Each cell has electrical properties and its own concomitant field. In 1940, researchers evaluated the polarity of an unfertilized egg. The egg was then fertilized, and it was observed that the brain and the spine formed on the axis of polarity that was present prior to fertilization. There is high-energy information outside of each cell that directs the activity of that cell. It is that information that interfaces with the electrochemical properties within each cell. The physical body is the product — the crystallization — of high-energy matter that is not visible.

Something exterior to the embryo precipitates the embryo's formation and rhythmic pulsations characteristic of the animal kingdom.

Developmental Information

We know that humans develop from one fertilized cell. The "genetic material" of the ova from which each of us developed was formed when our mothers themselves were fetuses. Our fathers' contributions to our genetic background, on the other hand, "was formed only two or three months prior to insemination." (Restak, p. 33)

Egg and sperm both have their own individual characteristics. They influence each other just by being in the universe. But the influence on each other isn't nearly as great as the positive and negative energy (or polarity) that draws them together. When the one-cell egg is fertilized, the cell divides to become two cells. Each daughter cell divides, and the process goes on until a complete human is formed. As cells divide, they differentiate to serve specific needs and to perform the complex interrelated variety of functions required for life and survival of a newborn.

With each cell division, the DNA (deoxyribonucleic acid) of that cell also divides. DNA is the blueprint that provides the information necessary for producing the final fully-developed product. DNA contains *all* of the information needed to form the finished whole. Unlike a half an orange that contains only half as much "meat" as the whole, the genetic information of the DNA is not "halved" when the cell divides. Remarkably, it retains its completeness in each segment.

DNA research has established that each cell contains all of the information necessary to construct a complete organism. Current wisdom advocates that cells differentiate into bone, muscle, nerve, or tissue cells through repression of specific genes in those cells. "Strange as it may seem," writes Guyton, "every nucleated cell of the body contains the same set of genes as those originally present in the fertilized ovum from which the body was formed." (Guyton, p. 33)

Just how differentiated cells know how to organize themselves to become a complete functioning entity is not known precisely. DNA contains information that allows cells to know how to perform their specialized function. Understanding that every cell contains the same "information" as every other cell of the body is significant in intrabody and interbody communication.

Each cell is a genetic replica of the original cell from which it developed. Each cell, no matter what function it may serve following differentiation, contains the same information as all other cells that came from the original cell. Some of this information is suppressed in order for specialization to take place. Cells form specific organs and carry out specific functions when particular elements of the DNA are suppressed. "Little is known concerning the manner in which genes are suppressed either permanently, as in differentiation, or temporarily. Each cell in the body, however, must contain all the information originally present in the fertilized egg. Yet, as is amply obvious, a fibroblast in the region of the big toe is incapable of producing insulin." (Orten & Neuhaus, pp. 118-119)

Although a connective tissue cell may not be able to produce insulin, differentiation of cells of a developing entity appears to be governed by the location in which the cell finds itself. Consider the lizard that loses its tail easily as a means of self-defense. After the tail is detached, a "strong organizing field" forms around the area where the tail is to regenerate. Dean Black, PhD, writes: "If you plant a tumor cell on the tail side of that point, the organizing field transforms it into a normal tail cell. But if you transplant it on the head side of the point, it remains a tumor cell and multiplies without direction." (Black, p. 46)

Black demonstrates cellular adaptation further by citing an experiment in which kidney cells of a rat were transplanted to the prostate gland "and the cells developed what the scientists called 'prostatic activity.'" (Black, p. 46) Cells take their cue from their surroundings.

Pondering these examples leads to considering whether bacteria could change from a symbiotic state to a pathogenic state just by changing the organizing field around them.

The question remains: what or where is the organizing "command post" that directs the function a cell will perform and the suppression of particular bits of DNA as a part of the grand plan of development? It isn't a voluntary activity in the mind of the mother. Ordinarily, several weeks of development have passed before the mother is aware that a new being is even present. The mother isn't in charge of the schedule of development. And the fetus certainly isn't in charge. The fetus is into the second week of development before the primitive streak, which is the precursor to the nervous system, begins to appear. (Langman, p. 50)

There is no conscious direction on the part of anyone that guides the pattern of development of a growing fetus. Yet every facet of the "production schedule" is carried out on time and in the proper sequence. An intelligence of some sort directs the activity of the genes of DNA, suppressing some and activating others. Since conscious thought is not involved, it is logical to infer that the motivation comes from another source.

Gerber proposes that, "It is highly likely that the spatial organization of the cells is ordered by a complex three-dimensional map of what the finished body is supposed to look like. This map or mold is the function of a bioenergetic field which accompanies the physical body." (Gerber, p. 51) Gerber cites Burr's findings that energy fields found around new sprouts of plants follow the form of the adult plant. (Gerber, p. 51)

Gerber uses the term "etheric body" to describe the field. He sees it as a "holographic template that carries coded information for the spatial organization of the fetus as well as a roadmap for cellular repair in the event of damage to the developing system." (Gerber, p. 51.) The electromagnetic field around the body provides the blueprint for organized fetal development.

By accepting this premise, we can see that as cells multiply, there is an association between their mass and the energy field that is around them. Since the egg is living matter, even before fertilization, there is electrical energy associated with it.

The ovum that is formed in a developing female contains informed energy from the parent ovum from which it was formed. This egg develops with all of the information contained in all of the energy of which it is constituted. In other words, the ova stored in the ovaries of a female fetus contain energy information accumulated from her mother and from her mother's mother. Energy information is both hereditary and contagious — it can be transmitted through genes and through electrons — genetically and "electron-ically."

Since this same energy has been circulating and interacting with other atomic and subatomic particles throughout time, it can be seen that all cells (comprised of energy-matter) are developed with the same energy-intelligence of all other cells. The energy that now comprises a heart cell may have at one time been a part of an ancient olive tree, or, just as easily, a cell of the iris of a baby's eye may contain the same energy that over the course of time was a part of a snake's digestive system, a rodent's ear, a hibiscus plant, and a Hawaiian fisherman. All energy is interlocked and all energy has been a part of many other forms of matter.

Following this thesis, it can be seen that the energy that forms all cells is the same energy that was included in the performance of functions of other systems. The "intelligence" that allowed the energy to be a part of other functions remains a part of the energy. As a result, all cells possess electron energy that carries the "intelligence" of the ages in addition to the intelligence of cellular DNA. Similarly, the energy that comprises fields around and within systems — energy that also has passed through the cycles of various systems — possesses the intelligence of the ages and the universe.

Burr found that "there was no significant change in the electro-metrics of the unfertilized [salamander] egg after fertilization. . . . apparently — in the salamander, at least — the electric field properties of the egg are established quite independently not only of the fact of fertilization but also of the plane of ingress of the sperm head into the egg." (Burr, p. 63) There are electrical properties associated not only with eggs and developing embryos, Burr also confirmed that there are electrical properties associated with all living adults.

For chiropractic, the crucial area of human embryonic development is not the complexities of gestation, but the genesis of the information that directs and guides the development and maintenance of all living creatures, fetal and adult. The same intelligence that guides the development of a fetus directs the repair of wounds and the replenishment of cells in the adult. A prime hypothesis of B.E.S.T. is that fields of electromagnetic energy are the prime movers of all life.

Cellular Communication

The human body lives or dies at the cellular level. If the cells are healthy and allowed to function optimally, the body is healthy. If the cells are neither healthy nor functioning at their best, the body dies, either slowly through protracted disease, or quickly through coronary "accidents," or other traumatic events.

Cells function properly when they live in a favorable internal environment. Cells remain healthy when they receive stimuli that prompt natural responses. The stimuli are generally considered to be of chemical or electrical origin. Chemical stimulation comes from substances introduced into the body. Some of the many chemical stimulants inflicted on the body of a typical citizen of a modern developed country include a variety of substances: appropriate nutrients (healthful, natural foods); alleged nutrients (highly refined or processed, unnatural foods); drugs (therapeutic or recreational); and environmental pollutants (industrial, agriculture, tobacco smoke) to name a few.

External electrical stimulation comes in the form of environmental impulses from such obvious sources as microwaves; high-tension wires; factory, office, and home equipment and appliances; electrical machinery; computers and TVs. Less obvious sources of electrical stimulation are the stimuli generated by thoughts and the influence of planetary and personal electromagnetic fields. No matter what the origin of the stimulus, cells — developing or mature — respond perfectly to each stimulus which they receive.

Electrical currents and their accompanying electromagnetic fields have an impact on the cells of developing life forms. This was illustrated in the early 1920's. In a study of regeneration by "a species related to the hydra," Elmer J. Lund of the University of Texas found that "a current strong enough to override the creature's normal polarity could cause a head to form where a tail should have reappeared." (Becker and Selden, pp. 82-83) Lund's work was followed in 1952 by G. Marsh and H.W. Beams who found that variations in current strength applied to a sectioned planarian resulted in a head forming at each end, or the head appearing where the tail should be and the tail where the head should be. "Marsh and Beams grew convinced that the animal's electric field was the morphogenetic organizing principle." (Becker and Selden, p. 84)

Electromagnetic fields are of at least equal importance in the development of embryos as are genes transmitted by the parents. "Genes give a cell power to adapt, but they don't guide it. The information that guides a cell comes from its context. This has been true from the moment we were conceived." (Black, p. 45)

One of the premises put forth in this book is that health — from the pre-fertilized egg until death — is dictated by two primary factors: (1) the presence or absence of defense physiology and (2) positive or negative forces of internal and external electromagnetic fields. Both of these factors influence the development of a fetus.

If the mother of an unborn child is in defense physiology (discussed later in this book) brought about by emotional or nutritional stress, the development of the child is affected. Likewise, if the internal and external electromagnetic fields of the mother are disrupted by negative thoughts, attitudes, and emotions, the development of the unborn child is affected. As is discussed throughout my writings, thoughts are the strongest single influence on health. Thoughts "make or break" the stability of an individual's personal electromagnetic field. When a pregnant woman's field is disrupted, the field controlling the development of cells, tissue, organs, and systems of her unborn child is also disrupted. When the energy projected by the mother (or any other individual) into her field resonates in harmony with that field and the universal field, health is mandated.

8

What Others Say About . . . Information And Communication

Chiropractic, since its inception in 1895, has viewed the body as an integrated unit that functions as a whole. Unlike some other health related fields that address individual effects of the body's function (symptoms), chiropractic acknowledged that the body is an integrated system. When one organ, tissue, or cell is affected, the whole body is affected.

During the 1980s, developments in B.E.S.T. convinced me that the principle function of the body is survival. In order for the body to survive as a system, every entity of the body — cells, tissue, organs, and structure — must communicate with all other entities. Internal communication is ordinarily thought of as involving nerves, synapses, hormones, and enzymes. While these are some of the vehicles through which the body communicates with its various members, the information to be transported by these vehicles originates in the energy received by the various members of the body. Information and communication comes through systems other than the sensory system.

A Czech scientist, Dr. Jan Brod, and his associates have demonstrated the physiologic characteristics of the fight-or-flight response in man in the laboratory setting. First, control measurements were made in a group of healthy young adults in a resting position. These subjects were then given a mental-arithmetic problem to solve: from a four-digit number like 1,194, subtract consecutive serial 17s. A metronome was set clicking in the background, and others around the subject made statements such as: "I did better than that. You're not doing very well." Then new measurements were taken of blood pressure, blood pumped by the heart, and blood pumped to the skeletal muscles. All had increased. . . . Other situations requiring behavioral adjustment also lead to the fight-or-flight response. All humans use the same basic physiologic mechanisms to respond to individually meaningful, stressful events. [Benson, pp 50-51. 1974]

S.P. Shchurin and two colleagues from the Institute of Automation and Electrometry have been awarded a special diploma by the USSR State Committee for Inventions and Discoveries for discovering that cells can "converse" by coding their messages in the form of a special electromagnetic ray.

The experimenters placed identical tissue cultures in two hermetically sealed vessels separated by a wall of glass, then introduced a lethal virus in one of the chambers which killed the colony of cells inside it. The second colony remained wholly unaffected. However, when they replaced the glass divider with a sheet of quartz glass and again introduced killing viruses to one of the colonies, the Soviet scientists were astonished to see that the second colony also met the same fate as the first, even though the viruses could not possibly have penetrated the barrier. . . .

Reports on this work in Moscow newspapers disclosed that, however fantastic it might seem, the ultraviolet radiation from the afflicted cells *carried information* encoded in the fluctuation in intensity which was somehow received by the second colony, just as words are transmitted and received in dots and dashes in the Morse code. [Tompkins and Bird, pp 212, 213. 1974]

I searched for cancer in the cell and I have found it in the form of a wrong coding in the brain. [Hamer. 1981]

There must be a way to receive information about external conditions, process it, and store it so that the

Information and Communication

data change the being's response to the same stimulus in the future. In other words, a sort of crude consciousness and memory must be present from the first. A life-form must also be able to sense damage and repair itself. Third, we can expect that it would show some sort of cyclic activity, perhaps tuned primarily to the circadian rhythm of the lunar day. Self-replication, one of the main requirements in the DNA -based theory, can be dispensed with. An organism that can fully heal itself is theoretically immortal. The criteria for life can be summarized as organization, information processing, regeneration, and rhythm. [Becker & Selden, p 257. 1985]

The invention of a better magnetometer has yielded definitive proof that's now widely acknowledged. Any electric current automatically generates a magnetic field around itself. Hence, as the perineural current conveys information in its fluctuations, it must be reflected by a magnetic field around the body, whose pulsing would reveal the same information. [Becker & Selden, p 239-240. 1985]

Variations in the current from one place to another in the perineural system apparently form part of every decision, every interpretation, every command, every vacillation, every feeling, and every word of interior monologue, conscious or unconscious, that we conduct in our heads. [Becker and Selden, p 241. 1985]

There no longer was any question that minute electrical phenomena, best understood on a semiconduction basis, accompanied, and more importantly, appeared to direct growth processes. By 1963 I was able to produce the first firm evidence for effects of external magnetic fields on the function of the central nervous system, and by the mid 1970's I was able to propose that the central nervous system was composed of two distinct but related systems. One, the more primitive, operating in a semiconducting fashion and utilizing actual electrical currents for the transmission of information, was related to the ancient acupuncture system. The other, the more evolutionarily recent, operated in the accepted fashion as a digital data transmission system that dealt mainly with such sophisticated processes as the special senses and motor integration. [Becker paper, p 77. 1986]

Wouter van Hoven. . .was careful, in the tests on plants that were deliberately maltreated, to take additional samples from other similar specimens nearby as controls. And he found, to his astonishment, that if these undamaged trees were anywhere near the injured ones, they showed a sympathetic increase in tannin concentration. A small hookthorn of the same size as the one that was thrashed and which stood over six feet away, showed a 42 percent increase in tannin after three hours. A silver oak ten feet away, produced 14 percent more tannin within an hour. Even the "weeping" of wattle was registered by two other trees within ten feet, which produced high concentrations of tannin soon after a student had belaboured their neighbour with his belt. . . . there are comparable conclusions in footnotes to the Washington study on alders and willows—and in another piece of recent research on polar and sugar maple trees in the woods of New Hampshire. [Watson, pp 50-51. 1986]

. . . because physics makes no distinction between particles in organic and inorganic matter, memory isn't something peculiar to brains. It can equally well be stored in a rock. As far as we know, rocks can't remember; but that doesn't mean that they don't hold a memory, or that we can never share it. In fact, there is a fair amount of evidence to suggest that this is precisely what some of us can do. [Watson, p 242. 1986]

Richard Dawkins, the Oxford biologist who drew attention to the tendency of genes to look after their own interests, was also responsible for identifying the 'meme'. He points out that words, phrases, fashions, theories and ideas are in effect non-physical genes, a

INFORMATION AND COMMUNICATION

kind of abstract DNA. They are very much alive, passing from brain to brain, propagating themselves by imitation. Looked at in this way, ideas have a reality of their own. They are realised physically, over and over again, as actual structures and processes in human nervous systems. And if Sheldrake is right, each time they form they gain strength and momentum, building up their morphogenetic fields, becoming an evolutionary force in their own right. [Watson, p 65. 1986]

Theodore Roszak, in his excellent book *Unfinished Animal*, notes that thought and emotion have been shown to produce distinct, and sometimes permanent, alterations in the body's organ systems. [Litvak & Senzee, p 132. 1986]

... immunological reactions may involve a learning or experiential factor in which antibodies are 'educated' to recognize specific antigens, with the resulting experience stored in memory. [Litvak & Senzee, p 133. 1986]

Possibly, the electric field was the vehicle for carrying design from the chromosome to the protoplasm. [Litvak & Senzee, p 130 . 1986]

Tissue growth and repair is the most dramatically evident example of duplication in the extant organism and, hence, the best argument for the template or "jelly mold." [Litvak & Senzee, p 131. 1986]

[Biophysicist Fritz A.] Popp sees electromagnetic waves in this context as quantum information carriers. Photons may carry the ciphers for all coded functions, including pathologies. Through their exchange (or that of any other energy quanta), the specific quantitative bursts of energy needed for DNA coding in the form are delivered. [Litvak & Senzee, p 132. 1986]

We have developed a detailed theoretical informational model which describes the manner in which specific low frequency waves and specific intensities affect the brain and central nervous system as well as the peripheral and parasympathetic nervous systems. Electrical impedance, piezoelectric response of collagen and the paramagnetic properties of heme are all involved in the electromagnetic informational content mechanisms of biological processes . . . . The reason the low intensity frequency fields affect biological processes is that they match the system's own informational system, and when properly matched, are interpreted as internally generated by the biological system itself. [Srinivasan, pp 208-209. 1988]

. . . we, as human organisms, are a series of interacting multidimensional subtle-energy systems, and . . . if these energy systems become imbalanced there may be resulting pathological symptoms which manifest on the physical/emotional/mental/spiritual planes. [From Introduction by Gabriel Cousens, M.D., Gerber p 28. 1988]

At the micro level, cells of living organisms display organizing principles which demonstrate that every piece contains the whole. . . . 'Phantom leaf' electrographs confirm that, within this energetic field pattern, every piece contains the information of the whole. [Gerber, p 63. 1988]

When human polymorphonuclear basophils, a type of white blood cell with antibodies of the immunoglobulin E (IgE) type on its surface, are exposed to anti-IgE antibodies, they release histamine from their intracellular granules and change their stain properties. The latter can be demonstrated at dilutions of anti-IgE that range from 1×10^2 to 1×10^{120}; over that range, there are successive peaks of degranulation from 40 to 60% of the basophils, despite the calculated absence of any anti-IgE molecules at the highest dilutions. Since dilutions need to be accompanied by vigorous shaking for the effects to be observed, transmission of the biological information could be related to the molecular organization of water. . . . we propose that none of the starting molecules is present in the dilutions beyond the Avogadro limit and that specific information must have been transmitted during the dilution/shaking process. Water could act as a 'template' for the molecule, for example by an infinite hydrogen-bonded network, or electric and magnetic fields. At present we can only speculate on the nature of the specific activity present in the highly diluted solutions. [Davenas, *et al.*, pp 816, 817. 1988]

Because the study of stress continues to produce hard evidence that emotions influence health, it is now inevitable that the findings of traditional medical research in this area will eventually merge with the principles of holistic health because both fields are discovering the same reality: Emotions exert the controlling influence upon the physical body. Even though the traditional medical community takes a more cautious approach in forming conclusions on this matter, the door, nevertheless, has been opened. [Shealy and Myss, p 7. 1988]

Within the unconscious domain, a person is able to control to some degree the function of involuntary processes associated with the autonomic or peripheral nervous system. This includes control over smooth muscles and glands which is achieved through subcortical brain structures. Control of normally unconscious processes creates distinctive results which can be used to demonstrate unusual states of mind. [Srinivasan, p 17. 1988]

. . . discoveries have been made that both the neuroendocrine and immune systems can produce identical substances (peptide hormones, or neuropeptides) that influence both neuroendocrine and immune activity. The two systems also share the same array of receptors with which these substances can interact and transmit their messages. Such evidence has led Dr. Blalock to believe that the central nervous system and immune system convey similar information to each other through such hormone signals.

These facts fit in with the last article written by the late Franz Inglefinger as editor of the *New England Journal of Medicine*, in which physicians were reminded that 85 percent of human illnesses are within the reach of the body's own healing system. Hence the importance of the expanding knowledge about the way mind and body can collaborate in meeting serious challenges. [Cousins, pp 37-38. 1989]

All sensory input, which begins in the brain, has its effect through the body. Few aspects of the brain are more fascinating or significant than the way it makes its registrations on the immune system. In this way, our thoughts can have an effect on health and our ability to turn back disease. Brain cells and immune cells are equipped for direct communication with one another.

These connections are so intimate that, according to Dr. Elena A. Korneva of the Institute for Experimental Medicine in Leningrad, USSR, stimulation to the front of the hypothalamus (which is involved in the calming of emotions and the body's ability to absorb nutrients for the healing process) *increases* the body's immune capability, which the back of the hypothalamus (which relates to stress, as in the "fight or flight" response), impairs the performance of disease-fighting cells in the immune system. Dr. Viktor M. Klimenko, a colleague of Dr. Korneva's, has shown that immune responses in turn cause chemical and electrical changes in the brain. [Cousins, pp 72-73. 1989]

One of the world's leading experts on behavioral medicine, Dr. Neal Miller of The Rockefeller University and Yale University, has emphasized that what is most significant about the placebo response is the proof it offers that thoughts or expectations can be converted into physiological reality. Dr. Miller's work makes a good case for the strategic and careful use of placebos in the treatment of patients.

That expectations can have a specific effect on the immune system has been demonstrated by Drs. Robert Ader and Nicholas Cohen of the University of Rochester, who have shown that the immune system can be trained, or "conditioned," to respond to a neutral stimulus (placebo), first reported in 1926 by S. Metal'nikov and V. Chorine of the Pasteur Institute in Paris. [Cousins, p 230. 1989]

Candace Pert... — then chief of the Brain Biochemistry section at the National Institute of Mental Health (NIMH) in Bethesda, Maryland — reacted the way scientists often do when things don't fit: they question the rigor of other people's science. 'I thought perhaps the work was sloppy, shoddy, didn't have the right controls,' she admits. 'When you can't fit it into your cosmos, it's a lot easier to think someone else is a slob.' Then Pert and her NIMH collaborator, Michael Ruff, began to find the same thing: certain white blood cells were equipped with the molecular equivalent of antennas tuned specifically to receive messages from the brain. [Hall. 1989]

... monocytes can settle down in the skin, lungs or brain and take up permanent residence as macrophages. Ruff's research shows that these cells, in motion or at rest, have enormous potential for sending and receiving biochemical messages. . . . Because of these cells' movement and informational dexterity, Pert and Ruff call them 'mobile synapses.' [Hall. 1989]

Ed Blalock, now at the University of Alabama at Birmingham, believes the immune system functions as a sensory organ, just like the eyes or nose: white blood cells recognize what he calls 'noncognitive stimuli,' such as bacteria and viruses, and these immune system cells influence behavior by unleashing a gush of powerful biochemicals. [Hall. 1989]

Would it be possible to tell which came first, the readiness potential or the conscious intention to act? ... Subjects did not decide to move [a hand or wrist] until three hundred and fifty milliseconds after the readiness potential had begun. In other words, their neurons were firing a third of a second before they were even conscious of the desire to act. [Libet. 1989]

My impression is that the strong conviction of the *validity* of a flash of inspiration (not 100 per cent reliable, I should add, but at least far more reliable than just chance) is very closely bound up with its aesthetic qualities. A beautiful idea has a much greater chance of being a correct idea than an ugly one . . . Hadamar (1945, p. 31) writes:

> ... it is clear that no significant discovery or invention can take place without the *will* of finding. But with Poincare, we see something else, the intervention of the sense of beauty playing its part as an indispensable *means* of finding. We have reached the double conclusion:
>
> that invention is choice
>
> that this choice is imperatively governed by the sense of scientific beauty.
>
> [Penrose, p 421. 1989]

Because of the fact that mathematical truths are necessary truths, no actual 'information,' in the technical sense passes to the discoverer. All the information was there all the time. It was just a matter of putting things together and 'seeing' the answer! [Penrose, p 428. 1989]

... some processing of visual information takes place in the retina itself, *before* the visual cortex is reached. (The retina is actually considered to be part of the brain!) [Penrose, p 387. 1989]

INFORMATION AND COMMUNICATION

We must 'see' the truth of a mathematical argument to be convinced of its validity. This 'seeing' is the very essence of consciousness. It must be present *whenever* we directly perceive mathematical truth. When we convince ourselves of the validity of Godel's theorem we not only 'see' it, but by so doing we reveal the very non-algorithmic nature of the 'seeing' process itself. [Penrose, p 418. 1989]

The first thing that is killed in the laboratory is the delicate web of intelligence that binds the body together. When a blood cell rushes to a wound site and begins to form a clot, it has not traveled there at random. It actually knows where to go and what to do when it gets there, as surely as a paramedic—in fact, more surely, since it acts completely spontaneously and without guesswork. Even if we break down its knowledge into finer and finer bits, looking for the secret in some minute hormone or messenger enzyme, we will not find a protein strand labeled 'intelligence,' and yet there is no doubt that intelligence is at work. [Chopra, pp 41-42 . 1989]

... mind is not confined to the brain by some neat division set up for our own convenience. Mind is projected everywhere in inner space. [Chopra, p 70. 1989]

A body that can 'think' is far different from the one medicine now treats. For one thing, it knows what is happening to it, not just through the brain, but everywhere there is a receptor for messenger molecules, which means on every cell. [Chopra, p 71. 1989]

... a cell's memory is able to outlive the cell itself. [Chopra, p 87. 1989]

Biologist Rupert Sheldrake (1987), ... favors the hypothesis that brains are, like TV's *tuning* devices, and the storage is outside the brain and body. This makes memory itself non-physical, an idea which receives strong support from research with non-ordinary states of consciousness (Stevenson, 1977; Grof, 1987). [Chamberlain, p 11. 1989]

... memory is possible without cells and memory endures while the cells do not. [Chamberlain, p 14. 1989]

In 1960, Kappers discovered that the primary nerves that serve the pineal originate not within the brain, but rather in the sympathetic nervous system (specifically in sympathetic cell bodies in the superior cervical ganglia). (cf. *The New Scientist*, July 25, 1985, and *Science News*, November 9, 1985.) [Shafica, p 103. 1989]

The term 'placebo' may thus be expanded from the textbook definition of an inactive or ineffective chemical agent, such as a 'sugar pill,' and applied to the *state of the patient's mind*. Taking this one step further, I believe that under the circumstance of such a profound belief, produced by any technique, the conscious mind of the patient is able to access the DC system of the body and produce healing. [Becker, p 101. 1990]

The ethical practitioners of minimal-energy techniques do not deceive their patients in this fashion. Instead, they tell patients from the start that they are going to cure *themselves* by learning techniques that will give them control over their own bodies. These practitioners are more like teachers than healers, guiding their patients into deeper self-knowledge and ability. This type of therapy must bring into play much more of the body's inherent control systems than the simple authoritarian placebo, and from that point of view it must be a more effective technique. The patients are in control of their own destinies. They make their own decisions and regulate their own healing, without being dependent on an authority figure. This may be a significant point in the success of these techniques, because developing this sense of independence, a feeling of control and self-determination, has been shown to significantly reduce the stress of a serious or life-threatening illness. [Becker, p 103. 1990]

9

Communication Through Fields

"Communication" can be viewed as a buzzword of the latter part of the twentieth century. Books, magazine and newspaper articles, and high-dollar seminars focus on teaching the gentle (and sometimes not so gentle) art of communication. Webster's Third New International Dictionary, Unabridged, lengthy definition of communication begins with: "the act or action of imparting or transmitting...."

Communication is ordinarily thought of as being between or among individuals. Communication in the B.E.S.T. sense takes place not only between individuals and within the matter that constitutes the body, but also between or among all living beings. In his fascinating book, *Beyond Supernature: A New Natural History of the Supernatural*, animal behavior expert, Dr. Lyall Watson describes what might be termed the great kudu murder committed by bushveld trees of the South African province of Transvaal. (Watson, pp. 46-50) Kudu are large antelopes that feed on vegetation. In the early 1980s, drought and fenced land reduced the forage material available to the kudu that, under ordinary circumstances, fed only lightly from individual trees. Reports of large numbers of kudu dying of starvation led researchers to investigate the cause. They found the stomachs of many of the dead kudu to contain leaves, yet the animals had obviously died of starvation. Investigations found that the leaves the kudu had been eating contained an inordinate amount of tannin, and that these chemical compounds had, in effect, tanned the intestine of the animals thereby effectively removing their nutrient assimilation capabilities. Further investigation revealed that the trees on which the animals were feeding showed low levels of tannins while they were undisturbed, but when the trees were molested by bludgeon-and belt-wielding students to mimic the abuse of a rough-foraging kudu, the tannin level of the leaves soared, in some instances as much as 282 percent. This process was a survival mechanism of the trees to protect themselves from destruction. Bitter tasting tannin produced by the leaves discouraged the kudu from continuing their meal at that particular tree.

However, an equally interesting response was found by unmolested control trees adjacent to the battered trees. The tannin level in the leaves of trees within a short distance, but without root contact between the two, also rose when their neighbors were attacked. The trees had communicated in some manner, without benefit of sensory apparatus with which we are familiar. One hypothesis to explain this phenomenon is that airborne chemical substances that initiated the rise in tannin were transferred between trees. A more likely explanation, albeit not as readily received by our chemicomechanical scientific authorities, is that of Innate communication through electromagnetic fields.

All matter and amalgamation of matter is incorporated within electromagnetic energy fields. The universe, the earth, all animals, vegetables, and minerals of the earth, and all of the molecules, atoms, subatomic particles that make up the objects of our world and beyond exist within their own fields.

Energy currents emanating from postnatal humans are measurable from outside the body. EEG readings of currents inside the brain, for example, are taken from the scalp rather than from inside the brain itself. EKG readings of cardiac currents are also taken externally rather than internally. These currents are energy, just as matter in motion is energy as exemplified in Einstein's noted equation $E=mc^2$.

B.E.S.T. also proposes that the electron field contains the wisdom and knowledge of the ages: past, present, and future. It is the internal electromagnetic field, made up of the billions of electrons associated with the atoms that make up the body, that serves as each individual's repository of intuitive knowledge. It is here that Innate resides. The information enmeshed in the internal fields of electron energy of each individual is the source of personal distinctiveness. Along with distinctive inherited genetic structure, each individual possesses distinctive inherited and accumulated field information. (This hypothesis is elaborated in the section "Embryogenesis.")

The information "imparted" within the body controls how the body functions. We have already touched on the fact that the central nervous system controls our voluntary actions and outward physical reactions, and the autonomic nervous system controls our internal physiological responses whether or not we are in defense physiology. These concepts that are the underpinning of the application of the Bio Energetic Synchronization Technique will be detailed in this book.

In the meantime, it is essential to understand that less obvious internal and external communication takes place through fields in and around the body.

A View Of The Unseen Fields

All matter is in motion in that the electrons included or comprising the matter are constantly in motion. Since all matter is made up of atomic particles including electrons, and since all electrons are constantly in motion, matter (including the constituent parts of the human body) is energy. The driving force of energy can also be seen as the driving force of cells. Conventional wisdom tells us that energy cannot be destroyed. It can be converted to another form, but it cannot be destroyed. Consequently, the driving force of energy cannot be destroyed, otherwise energy would be destroyed.

The impetus of energy always functions perfectly; it informs (provides form and character) energy.

Within the past decade or two, the energy field concept has been moving out of the realm of metaphysics into the scientific arena. "Bioplasma body," "L-Fields," "M-Fields," "corona discharge," are just some of the names attached to fields. State-of-the-art technology now provides means by which fields can be measured and photographed. Holographic images provide visual representations of heretofore unseen fields recorded by the use of a laser beam. This beam is the same coherent light used in fiberoptic telecommunications and laser eye surgery. Holographic images afford a unique three-dimensional view of an object. A unique aspect of holographic images is that the image of the original object (Gerber uses the example of an apple) can be cut into sections — halves, quarters, 64ths, or smaller — and when viewed "under the illumination of laser light, a smaller, yet intact, whole apple can be seen." (Gerber, p. 47)

Holographic pictures not only capture a three-dimensional representation of the subject, but any segment of the holographic image reveals a representation of the whole. The holographic principle that "every piece contains the whole" gives new meaning to the chiropractic tenet of "above down, inside out." This "each part contains the whole" concept (the basis for cloning frogs), is not new to scientific thought.

Holography is perhaps most widely recognized by the name "Kirlian photography." In the early 1940s, the Russian researcher, Semyon Kirlian, investigated "measuring changes in the energy fields of living systems." (Gerber, p. 53) He and Burr were on the same mission of measuring electrical fields of the body but they were taking different routes. Burr produced statistical data while Kirlian produced "visual characteristics of an electrical corona." (Gerber, p. 53) Evidence is mounting of the validity of what Gerber terms "a holographic energy body."

The significance of holography is twofold: it renders observable the energy activity around the body which is ordinarily unobservable; and it emphasizes that each part of the body is a representation of the whole. The holographic phenomenon supports the concept that all areas of the body are affected when any area of the body is affected.

A video presentation has recently become available that depicts visual representation of the external fields surrounding the body. Several subjects are used to demonstrate that the fields exist and that fields change shape and "intensity" according to the activities of the individual. The field is active and extends several feet from the subject. Fields around adults and children are seen to fluctuate. In some instances, an individual's field is unevenly dispersed in that the width of the corona is narrow around certain areas of the body and wide around other areas.

Field volume appears to change. When a person who is shown eating healthful "living" food, such as fresh fruit, switches to eating highly processed "dead" food, the field that had been vibrant and robust subsides and becomes less vibrant and narrower than it was under the influence of "live" food.

This demonstration illustrates a form of internal communication since activities taking place inside the body affect the field outside the body. The body continuously communicates with its field. How this field communication occurs is, at this point, subject to conjecture only. Authors from a variety of disciplines offer their own explanations. The B.E.S.T. hypothesis holds that the fields and communication with and within fields is associated with subatomic electron activity.

Electron Information

We know that electromagnetic forces exist just as we know electrons exist. Yet neither can be captured and held static for analysis. We cannot "observe" electromagnetism or electrons. We can observe the effects of electromagnetic forces, and we can observe the electron field.

As electrons move among atoms, ions, and molecules, the electron energy takes different shapes, and the associated fields are altered. Each time an electron is incorporated or lost from an atom, molecule or ion, the fields that had surrounded the individual entities are changed. When a hydrogen atom loses an electron, the energy field around the newly formed ion is changed and the energy field around the electron is changed. The energy, or "information," contained in the original fields is retained by the former field and incorporated into the new field. Atomic and subatomic energy fields constantly overlap and integrate as molecular components move about in tightly packed areas. If energy "information" contained in one field is replicated in another field in the course of forming and re-forming atoms, molecules, and ions, all information is contained in all fields. "Information" is universal.

Gerber tells us, "there is consciousness in all aspects of matter, from the human level on down to the atomic level.... All matter, even at the subatomic level, is formed of tiny drops of frozen light—a kind of focused mini-energy field. There is consciousness in this basic energy unit. It is the prime ingredient forming the basic building blocks of the universe. Its basic energetic properties may be seen reflected in all aspects of creation. All particularizations of this energy, such as atoms or even electrons, have some rudimentary form of consciousness, albeit highly different from what one considers as human consciousness." (Gerber, pp. 350, 351)

"Information" includes all present, past, and as yet untapped knowledge necessary to the functioning of organized systems of the universe, planets, creatures, and cells. Information directs the formation and maintenance of living creatures. Each living creature develops through the direction of universal information. This information, as we shall see, knows neither language nor time as man knows them. It is ever-present, yet different species utilize different aspects of the same information.

The electron field is observable but ethereal. B.E.S.T. postulates that incorporated into the subatomic field of electrons is "information," or "consciousness," pertaining to all matter with which the electron has ever been associated. "Information" is magnetic energy, and energy is information in expression.

Fields Of Information

The physicalness of a living body is the raw template that acts as a receiver of universal information. The embryo of a dog is a different template from that of a human embryo, however, both have access to the same energy information. The availability of energy information is universal — the reception of the energy information is species-specific. Working with the same information, the saliva of a dog is pH 4.0 while the saliva of a human is (or should be) pH 8.0.

Fields of information are interrelated, contiguous, overlapping, and meshed. Information is transmitted between and among fields incessantly. How we react *with* field information is more important than how we react *to* sensory information. As we respond, we become a different entity — a different receiver. As soon as we receive and utilize information, we become a different system. The updated system transmits information that is different from the information of a millisecond earlier. Transmission of information through fields constitutes creation. Through unceasing, integrated alterations in energy information fields, man (and all other living creatures) is in a continuous process of both evolution and creation.

As fields converge and diverge, they change. Just as a person who gains additional information is "different" from the person he was before the information was acquired, so fields are different with each interfield contact. There is an inter-reaction between the electron fields of the physical body and the fields within and about the body, and an interrelation with those fields and the universe. When man becomes sick, communication with his external field is impaired and, as will be discussed in another chapter, he responds to the information of his own field rather than to that field that was responsible for his creation. Defense physiology is a manifestation of interference in communication with the creating field around the body.

Since all things in the universe are made up of all things in the universe, then all things in the universe know all things. Keep in mind that this knowledge is subconscious. The subconscious mind is filled with information that is inaccessible to the conscious mind until relevant "lessons" are learned to release the information to the conscious level.

Although all things are known, the information available to one individual is different from that available to another. Even brothers, sisters, or identical twins have enough variation in the substance of the information available to them to create unique entities.

An analogy illustrating how information differentiates apparently similar beings can be drawn from a hypothetical exercise in analyzing two video or audio tapes; one tape has sounds recorded on it, the other tape is "clean." Laboratory analysis of the structure and components of both tapes will reveal no differences in their physical properties. However, one contains information and the other does not. In the same way, analysis of the electromagnetic fields in and around the body will reveal given strengths, but current instrumentation cannot analyze or detect the information contained in those fields. Only when the body "plays back" the information recorded in the fields around it through manifestation of health, disease, or a high-level of communication can the information accumulated in the fields be understood.

Unlimited Interrelationships

In order to describe the influence of electromagnetic fields on physiological activity, it is essential to acknowledge the interrelationship of all matter and systems.

There is growing acceptance of the holistic concept not only with regard to maintaining the health of the body but also to the interrelatedness of the body with the immediate environment. This interrelatedness extends from the body itself to the individual's surroundings, the ecology of the world, and electromagnetic forces of the universe. The mutuality of the universe and all things in it was concisely implied by the noted English astronomer and mathematician Sir Arthur Eddington: "When the electron vibrates, the universe shakes."

The fact that instrumentation has not yet been devised to monitor the effects of electromagnetic forces on health speaks more to the limitations of man's cognitive knowledge than to the inappropriateness of consideration of these forces.

Our inability to measure "diffuse states of matter-energy" was addressed in 1980 by F.W. Cope of the Biochemistry Laboratory, Naval Air Development Center in Warminster, Pennsylvania, writing for *Physiological Chemistry and Physics* (Vol 12, No. 4, 1980, 349-355).

> The evidence now available suggests that all objects, and especially living objects, contain, are surrounded by, and interact with clouds of diffuse matter-energy at least some of which has been radiated to the earth from the sun. I describe these clouds as composed of diffuse relativistic superconducting plasma. Relativistic considerations lead to the conclusion that it is impossible for an *outside* observer to measure most physical parameters *inside* that plasma system. Nevertheless, the system can be expected to make its presence known by effects it produces on physical parameters outside itself, and these *outside* effects should be measurable by an *outside* observer. Such outside effects may be accentuated by applied high voltages, as in Kirlian photography, and may reveal themselves by synchronization of electromagnetic oscillations in adjacent molecules resulting in laser action with observable electromagnetic emissions. (Cope, p. 350)

Although the expansion of concepts of health care to include other- than-observable elements may appear to be combining the realms of physics and metaphysics, it is the contention of the author that the two must be considered jointly in order to best serve the health care needs of the patient. Human beings are composites of tangible and intangible factors. Neither can be considered in isolation if the best interest of the complete person is to be served.

Communicating Change

Electrons are continuously mobile. It is through their movement that molecules and ions are formed and reformed. Since electrons may be unique in their characteristic of being both wavelike and particulate, electron energy can be seen as "circulating" through the universe in the form of light and through matter in the universe in the form of particles as well as through the diffuse superconductive plasma about which Cope writes.

Electron-containing atomic and molecular matter as we know it — everything from the ingredients of the earth itself to styrofoam to the human body — is subject to continuous change. Each change is a response to a stimulus. Although some of the change processes may be so slow and of such duration that man has not yet been in existence long enough to witness it, nonetheless, evidence points to the consistency of change. In animate creatures, the change is obvious — the cycle of birth, maturation, and death. For example, a plant. Throughout its life cycle, the plant changes. Cells of the seed reproduce, differentiate, mature, function, and die.

Yet the energy that was once plant material does not die. The electrons live on. Electrons that once were a part of an ear of corn may be incorporated into the soil if the ear falls to the ground and is left to decay, or they may be consumed by an animal or a person and be assimilated into a cell of that organism. Eventually, the host organism dies or is discarded and the electron is on the move again ready to be assimilated into another form of matter.

In each of these instances, the electron energy field persists. We might hypothesize that the field in which electrons orbit , rather than being "space," is in reality matter at a frequency higher than we can as yet monitor. Even more important, these spaces can be seen as holding the key to communication among cells of the body, between subconscious minds, and with the universe.

10

What Others Say About...
The Influence Of
Fields And Currents

If we accept the existence of energy fields in and around the body and that subtle forms of energy affect living systems, we must then accept that electromagnetic fields in and around the body influence the functioning of the body just as do all elements which constitute the environment in which the body functions.

... instruments have found what [Dr. Burr] and Dr. Northrop postulated over thirty years ago. Countless experiments have demonstrated that the electric fields they discovered serve basic functions, controlling growth and morphogenesis, maintenance and repair of living things. Naturally, these differ from the alternating-current electric output of the brain and heart, as well as from the epiphenomenal skin-resistance, serving rather as an electronic matrix to keep the corporal form in shape. (From: Ravitz, Leonard J. , M.S., M.D., F.R.S.H., "Electro-Magnetic Field Monitoring of Changing State-Function Including Hypnotic States," published in *Journal of American Society of Psychosomatic Dentistry and Medicine*, Vol. 17, No. 4, 1970.) [Burr, p 156. 1972]

Using micro-pipettes filled with salt solution and connected to the voltmeter we found different voltage gradients across different axes of the [frog] eggs. We marked the axis of the largest voltage gradient with spots of Nile blue sulphate and later found, as the eggs developed, that the frog's nervous system always grew along the axis with the highest voltage gradient. This was an indication that the field is primary—the matrix that shapes the living form. [Burr, p 61. 1972]

With the co-operation of the Connecticut Agricultural Experiment Station, it became possible to study the electrical patterns in several pure and hybrid strains of sweet corn.... The strains differ considerably in genetic constitution and in the degree of hybrid vigour shown in crosses between them. . . . In this material, therefore, we had four stable pure strains of significantly different properties with which to correlate electrical patterns.... A statistical analysis shows that the mean potential measured between the attached end of the corn kernel and its opposite pole gave highly significant results.... Aside from the generally different mean, however, the most striking finding was a very great difference between the mean of the single gene mutant and the parent stock. It is remarkable that the change of a single gene in the parent stock should produce such profound and significant change in the over-all pattern of the voltage difference. The conclusion seems to be inescapable that there is a very close relationship between the genetic constitution and the electrical pattern. [Burr, p 71. 1972]

The human body is under the influence of the earth's magnetic field and is keeping some sort of balance relationship with it. However, under modern day living conditions, the effect of this field has decreased. Consequently, we can assume that for a certain human body, this lack of magnetism has caused some abnormalities. For this reason, by the external application of a magnetic field to the human body to supplement this deficiency, such abnormal conditions can be improved. In other words, I feel that there is a direct relationship between the decrease in the earth's magnetic field acting on the human body and the improvement of abnormal conditions of the human body by the application of magnetic fields. [Nakagawa, p. 1. 1976]

The Influence Of Fields And Currents

The symptoms of the [magnetic field deficiency] syndrome are: 'Stiffness' of the shoulders, back and scruff of the neck, uncertain lumbago, chest pains for no specific reason, habitual headache and heaviness of the head, dizziness and insomnia for uncertain reasons, habitual constipation, general lassitude, etc. [Nakagawa, p.1. 1976]

In other words, it is a syndrome in which no objective pathological findings can be noticed from routine physical and clinical examinations, but in which the subjective symptoms persist and are hard to improve, resisting various treatments but responding to the application of a magnetic field. An unbalanced autonomic nervous system or part of such might be included in this syndrome. [Nakagawa, p. 1. 1976]

The earth's magnetic field is of course a stationary magnetic field working constantly on the human body. [Nakagawa, p. 4. 1976]

It is clear that an electric change will occur when a magnetic field is applied to the human body, but this is not an insertion of electrical energy into the body it is only a conversion of a part of the motion energy of the body fluid into electrical energy through the medium of a magnetic field. Therefore, we cannot consider it as an insertion of energy as the energy of the magnetic field is much smaller than other physical phenomena used for therapy today. For this reason, we feel that if such an energy change is produced by applying a magnetic field constantly to the human body, some change will occur in the body. [Nakagawa, p. 5. 1976]

Recent explorations with a vibrating probe show that a wide variety of developing systems drive strong steady electrical currents through themselves. . . . Moreover, substantial evidence indicates that these currents—or at least some of them—act back to affect development. [Jaffe, p 569. 1979]

In addition to indicating zones of junctional disruption, these strong outward currents may well act back to control, to further, or even to organize development. [Jaffe, p 570. 1979]

Bassett's coils are so simple to operate that astronauts may use them in space to prevent what NASA officials commonly refer to as astro-osteoporosis. Astronauts' bones become thin and brittle owing to a loss of calcium. Over prolonged space missions, the condition worsens. . . . But astro-osteoporosis is not a disease. In fact, it is a remarkable adaptation to life in zero gravity. 'The astronauts produced less bone,' says Bassett, 'because they didn't need big, heavy bones in the weightlessness of space. Their bone was under less mechanical stress. Hence, it did not generate the normal electrical voltages that help maintain bone formation.' The coils, he believes, should counteract what would otherwise be a superior adaptation to permanent residence in space. [McAuliffe, p 98 . 1980]

Lately, . . . buoyed by reports that electric currents, generated within embryos themselves, guide the development of species as diverse as brown seaweeds, frogs, insects, and chicks. Lionel Jaffe of Purdue University says, "We knew from physiology that the electrical machinery was there; living cells have these powerful batteries in their membranes. If they were distributed unevenly, they would lead to electric currents that might affect cell processes." [Marx, 1147. 1981]

Using the vibrating probe, Jaffe and Nuccitelli found that the fertilized *Pievetia* egg, In Nuccitelli's words, "drives an ion current through itself as early as we can measure, which is about 30 minutes after fertilization. . . . The inward current region always predicts the germination site." [Marx, p 1147. 1981]

The Influence Of Fields And Currents

... Robinson recently found that embryonic frog nerves, when grown in culture under the influence of an electric field, grow toward the negative pole of the field, even turning through large angles to do so. In addition, the field stimulates the growth of greater numbers of nerve projections. . . . "It is tempting to speculate" he [Robinson] says, "that embryonic currents are guiding the nerve growth." [Marx, p 1149. 1981]

Under the assumption that the BCEC [Biologically Closed Electric Circuits] systems represent a physiological transport mechanism which influences normal functions, including healing, it seams reasonable to speculate that *artificial activation of BCEC systems offers the possibility of enhancing healing.* [Nordenstrom, p 9. 1983]

... an external magnetic field moving in relation to BCEC circuits will produce a flow of current in the BCEC channels. *The BCEC system then can be seen to act as a receptor for external electromagnetic forces.* Such forces, both man-made and natural, are parts of our normal surroundings and within certain limits evidently well tolerated. [Nordenstrom, p 10. 1983]

The movements of collections of ions (ionars) in a closed circuit will of necessity induce magnetic fields in surrounding tissue. Conversely, motion of an external magnetic field in relation to BCEC channels will induce electric transports in these channels. BCEC systems can be expected therefore also to act as receptors for surrounding manmade as well as natural electromagnetic fields. [Nordenstrom, p 171. 1983]

These correlations, [Burr and Northrop] suggest, depend on interactions between particles and fields at the atomic level. According to this theory, 'the pattern or organization of any biological system is established by a complex electrodynamic field, which is in part determined by its atomic physiochemical components and which in part determines the behavior and orientation of these components.' In this theory the characteristic relationships of the elements of any biological system are a function of the field of the system. [Nordenstrom, p 318. 1983]

The *spontaneous healing of fractures may proceed by an analogous mechanism. Initially, callus may be formed during an acid injury phase. Not until the produced matrix turns into an electronegative phase will calcium ions be attracted and precipitate, leading to firm healing of the fracture.* [Nordenstrom, p 325. 1983]

An acceptance of BCEC systems leads to the necessary conclusion that these systems should act as receptors for moving external electromagnetic fields. [Nordenstrom, p 335. 1983]

Reports ... indicate that calcified tissues are not only influenced by applied magnetic fields but that tissues themselves exhibit magnetic properties.
[Papatheofanis, p 251. 1984]

Although an understanding of the effects of magnetic fields on biological systems is of critical practical importance in assessing occupational and therapeutic risk, an appreciation of the interaction of biological systems with magnetic fields should provide important insight into how nature operates at the most fundamental physical levels. [Papatheofanis, p 254. 1984]

Twenty-four male Lewis's white rats, aged twelve weeks at the beginning of the experiments, served as subjects.... In twelve pairs of animals, the left common peroneal nerve was sectioned and immediately sutured just above the level of the knee joint.... Half of each operative group received 400 electromagnetic pulses per second at 4 peak power (400-4) daily for fifteen minutes and sham treatment of the same duration was

The Influence Of Fields And Currents

given to the other half. The observer was unaware of which of the two machines was active, i.e. producing a double blind technique.... In animals whose nerves were sectioned and repaired but without PEMF treatment, the paralysed limb was first used for locomotion and grooming at the 21st post-operative day. In PEMF treated animals, it was first used in locomotion and grooming on the *12th* post-operative day. In untreated animals, the toe spreading reflex had not re-appeared in animals sacrificed at 3 ½ days, one week or at two weeks, but first became positive on the *21st* day in animals surviving to that time. In four pairs of treated and surviving animals, it was positive on the *12th* day in three pairs and on the *14th* day in the fourth (Mean = 12.5 days ± 1.0 S.D.). [Raji, pp 105-106. 1984]

Recently a group under Indian biophysicist Sarada Subrahmanyam reported that the human EEG not only responded to the micropulsations [of the earth's electromagnetic field], but responded differently depending on which way the subject's head was facing in relation to the earth's field. Oddly enough, however, the head direction had no effect if the subject was a yogi. [Becker and Selden, p. 249. 1985]

There is, insisted Burr, a veritable 'life-field' which holds the shape of an organism just as a mould determines the shape of a pie or a pudding.... [Watson, p 93. 1986]

We are, it seems, electric animals with sensitive magnetic minds, caught up in a web of electromagnetic influence. And it is somewhere in this energetic web that we have to look for the impetus that made us conscious and gave us the ability to knit ourselves into such a[n electropollution] tangle. [Watson, p 103. 1986]

We should also bear in mind that electromagnetic radiation can bypass the sense organs and affect the cells of the body directly. Dr. W. Ross Adey, head of UCLA's Brain Research Institute, has shown that a weak, pulsating electric charge applied to metal plates several inches on either side of a person's head can significantly alter the ability to estimate time, especially if the pulsations are in the range of seven cycles a second. Experiments of this type on cats and monkeys have revealed changes in brain chemistry and electrical activity as well as time sense. [Leonard, p 50-51. 1986]

The electric field, ... was an *electronic matrix to keep the corporeal form in shape.* Tissue growth and repair in all organisms, as well as birth and death themselves, are regulated by L-fields, according to Ravitz. He stressed the difference between these template fields and other, organ-associated electricity such as the alternating-current output of the brain and heart and epiphenomenal skin resistance. [Litvak & Senzee, p 131. 1986]

It will be recalled that Dr. Burr carried out experiments mapping the electrical fields around developing salamander embryos. Through his research, he discovered that an electrical axis developed in the unfertilized salamander egg which corresponded to the future orientation of the brain and central nervous system in the adult organism. The creation of such an electrical axis or wave guide in the unfertilized egg suggests that some type of directional energy field cooperates with and provides spatial orientation to the rapidly dividing and migrating cells of the newly forming embryo. Burr also discovered that in plant seedlings, the contour of the electrical field surrounding the new sprouts followed the shape of the adult plant. If we combine our knowledge of Kirlian photography's ability to capture the phantom leaf phenomenon with the aforementioned data, we come to the conclusion that *the spatial organization of growth from embryogenesis through adulthood is guided by a holographic energy-field template known as the etheric body.* [Gerber, p 125. 1988]

Abnormal structuring in the etheric template eventually leads to disruptive changes at the cellular level of the physical body. Therefore, physical illness may begin first at the etheric level before physical cellular changes have even started. [Gerber, p 82. 1988]

In mammals, the pineal gland (Semm *et al.*, 1980) is a light-sensitive, time-keeping organ in which the cell activity is affected by magnetic field pulses of the order of the strength of the geomagnetic field. It is possible that the pineal gland in higher animals and man may have shifted its electromagnetic sensitivity away from a predominantly visible-light sensitivity, characteristic of the submammalian vertebrates. [Smith & Best, p 44. 1989]

It is one of the universal miracles of nature that huge assemblages of particles, subject only to the blind forces of nature, are nevertheless capable of organising themselves into patterns of cooperative activity. [Davies p 4. 1989]

According to Ravitz, electromagnetic fields act as determiners of biological activity, rather than as epi-phenomena, patterning the nervous system and regulating every component part of it from within and without; they define living matter in terms of four-dimensional time-space and energy. [Smith & Best, p 38. 1989]

No clear boundary exists between the organism's metabolically maintained electromagnetic fields and those of its geophysical environment. Professor Frank A. Brown, Jr (1906-83). [Smith & Best, p 35. 1989]

... magnetic and electromagnetic fields have energy, can carry information, and are produced by electrical currents. When we talk about electrical currents flowing in living organisms, we also imply that they are producing magnetic fields that extend outside of the body and can be influenced by external magnetic fields as well. [Becker, 1990 p 69]

It may be a little disconcerting to know that we, and all other living things, are surrounded by a magnetic field extending out into space from our bodies, and that the fields from the brain reflect what is happening in the brain. The implications of this are enormous, . . . [Becker, 1990, p 70]

If we had the right amount of electrical current, in less than an hour we could watch one red corpuscle change from a cell filled with hemoglobin containing a small, shriveled-up nucleus, to a cell with no hemoglobin and a large active nucleus. . . . The results were of fundamental importance in bringing about the present scientific revolution. They clearly showed that the activities of living cells could be markedly influenced only by certain levels of extremely small electrical current. [Becker, 1990, p 70]

The data obtained in the past few years indicate very clearly that we must now include the Earth's normal geomagnetic field as an environmental variable of great consequence when we deal with the basic functions of living things. In my opinion, this knowledge is probably the single most important discovery of the century. It provides us with a key to the mechanisms by which all electromagnetic fields produce biological effects, and it may enable us to determine more accurately the risks involved in our technological uses of such fields. [Becker, 1990, p 247]

11

Rhythmic Patterns Of Life

Our universe and all that is in it marches to rhythmic patterns. Planets orbit in systematized patterns; the moon follows its course around the earth according to a prescribed time pattern; the seasons of the year conform to a cyclical sequence; tides ebb and flow on schedule; and man follows predictable phases of growth and development between conception and death. Our world functions in orderly (but sometimes clandestine) sequential rhythmic patterns. In like manner, the human physiology functions rhythmically. The pulse of life is in and around us.

Throughout life, even the atoms that make up our bodies engage in what has been termed life's "biodance" of continuous creation and re-creation of cells and organisms. Atoms circulate. They move from one entity to another. Hair and fingernails grow and "re-create" themselves, broken bones knit, and lacerated tissue heals. Less obvious is the "re-creating" activity of internal organs. "Every body structure has its own rate of reformation: the lining of the stomach renews itself in a week; the skin is entirely replaced in a month; the liver is regenerated in six weeks." Every atom of the body is replaced every five years. (Dossey, p. 74) None of us is the same person we were five years ago, although most of us are immediately recognizable by a friend who has not seen us in the interim.

Even more startling than realizing that each individuals' exterior and interior is in a constant state of flux is to understand, that our genes, the bedrock of the individuality, constantly change. Dossey tells us that the DNA molecule is no more fixed than is any other molecule. "Our restless genes are continually renewing themselves, exchanging bits and pieces for replacement parts. ...over a period of months our entire genetic structure is renewed." (Dossey, p. 73)

Of course, although the structure may be renewed, the pattern is not. What a confused society we would have if the pattern of our replaced genes altered during each change. Our person, reflected by our physiognomy, would be fluid. We wouldn't be able to recognize even our own parents or children if we hadn't seen them in a while.

We are constantly recreating ourselves and evolving by atoms we take into our bodies in the process of eating and breathing. Each time we breathe, we inhale atoms that have been coursing through the earth's atmosphere, entities, and other living creatures. Murchie calculated that "each breath you breathe must contain a quadrillion (10^{15}) atoms breathed by the rest of mankind within the past few weeks and more than a million atoms breathed personally sometime by each and any person on Earth." (Dossey, p. 77) Not only does mankind share the same turf, "we are all partners in the biodance." (Dossey, p. 77) We share in the substance and rhythm of life.

Physiological Pulsations

Pulsations are observable in human organisms at (and even before) conception. Cardiac pulses are obvious. Yet other, less apparent, rhythmical patterns have been found. The sources of some pulses are recognized, others are not. Various researchers cite the presence of pulsations. Mountcastle reports: "Recordings from the surface of the cerebellum take the form of low-voltage sinusoidal waves recurring at rates of 100 to 300/sec. Superimposed on them is a continuous background of smaller fluctuations at frequencies of 1,000 to 2,000/sec. The origin of the latter type of activity is not established." (Mountcastle, p. 1775)

And, Guyton states, "Some neuronal pools emit output signals continuously even without excitatory input signals. At least two different mechanisms theoretically can cause this effect: (1) intrinsic neuronal discharge and (2) reverberatory signals." (Guyton, p. 569) He goes on to explain: "Many neuronal circuits emit rhythmic output signals—for instance, the rhythmic respiratory signal originating in the reticular substance of the medulla and pons.... Many rhythmic signals are postulated to result from reverberating signals or successive reverberating circuits that feed excitatory or inhibitory signals from one to the next. However, many other more complex mechanisms could also be responsible for rhythmic signals." (Guyton, p. 569)

Four physiological pulsations, specifically of the brain, were noted by Magoun: (Magoun, pp. 23-24)

1. A pulsation which is synchronous with cardiac contractions.
2. A pulsation which coincides with respiratory pressure changes associated with inhalation and exhalation.
3. A wave not related to either heart rate or respiration but one which constantly maintains its own cycle.
4. An undulating pulsation which has not been identified.

Magoun cites references to pulsations by other researchers: Woolley and Shaw noted "rhythmical contractions of the oligodendroglial cells of the neuroglia in the central nervous system," and "Hyden and others showed that glial cells, grown in tissue culture, pulsate continuously." (Magoun, p. 24) The author goes on to confirm that "it is possible to feel rhythmic impulses on the human skull exhibiting an average of 10-14 cycles per minute in normal adults. This requires very gentle proprioceptive palpation. Corroborative recordings have been made electronically with definite separation from the pulse and respiration." (Magoun, p. 25)

A recent study of "synchronised spontaneous activity (SSA)" was performed by Barone, et al. This Italian team, using a neuromagnetic technique, found that "the brain reacts to sensory stimulation producing oscillatory responses that persist in the silent period [following stimulation]." The researchers concluded that "SSA are actually the superposition of two, possibly distinct, generators." (Barone, et al, pp. 71-76)

B.E.S.T. research and clinical experience have found that subcutaneous pulses appear on or near the spinal column in conjunction with areas of tenderness (not pain) of which the patient may be unaware until palpation. For the patient who presents with legs uneven in length, these pulses are asynchronous with pulses at other areas of tenderness. Slight tactile pressure on two areas of equal tenderness usually brings the pulses into synchronization within a minute. As the pulses become synchronized, the tenderness of one or both points diminishes, then disappears. Electromagnetic homeostasis is restored, pain subsides, and the body is again able to perform its self-healing functions. The paradigm for the most efficient and effective technique for locating areas of tenderness has been developed through clinical B.E.S.T. research and experience.

B.E.S.T. procedures utilize physiological pulses to communicate directly with the sensory system. Communication is established through digital palpation of tender areas that are characterized by small edematous nodules, many of which may be found on and around the spine. Although these nodules have not been identified, they could be viewed as being similar to Iggo dome receptors made up of "free (nonencapsulated) nerve ending" Merkel's discs. Guyton describes these receptors: "Merkel's discs are often grouped together in a single receptor organ called the Iggo dome receptor, which projects upward against the underside of the epithelium of the skin,... This causes the epithelium at this point to protrude outward, thus creating a dome. . . . the entire group of Merkel's discs is innervated by a single large type of myelinated nerve fiber (type AB). Each dome receptor has a diameter averaging only 0.2 mm, and these receptors are extremely sensitive. They probably play an important role in localizing touch sensations to the specific areas of the body." (Guyton, p. 581)

Although Iggo dome receptors are minute in size, they include cytoplasm and Schwann cells that could enlarge the area to the size discernable on palpation. "In the PNS [peripheral nervous system], the neurolemma cell has an outer collar of cytoplasm which loosely interdigetates in the nodal region with the outer collar of the adjacent neurolemma cell." (Noback & Demarest, p. 61) This hypothesis could account for both the spongy nature and extreme sensitiveness of the nodules utilized in B.E.S.T. adjustments.

Anatomical Pulsations

Pulsations are observable in human organisms at (and even before) conception. Both the sperm and egg pulsate independently prior to union. Following unification, the fertilized egg, devoid of developed nervous system or cardiovascular system, establishes its own rhythm. Pulsations of the heart are obvious. Yet other, less apparent, rhythmical patterns have been found. As noted earlier, the source of some pulsations are recognized, others are not.

B.E.S.T. diagnostic techniques involve the physical manifestations of electromagnetic impulses detectable in the human body as subtle yet distinct pulses. Although the "living" quality of the network of physiological systems and organs is unidentified as to the relationship to health and disease, it can be discerned through these subtle pulses.

Also over a decade ago, a specific method of palpation to detect pulsations of the scalp was described in *Osteopathic Annals*. The procedure called for placing the pads of two fingers "directly over the painful suture area.... The exact location can easily be determined in a few seconds with an extremely light palpatory touch." The purpose of this treatment was to relieve the symptoms of an autogenic headache, yet it aptly describes the epidermal pulsations utilized in the application of B.E.S.T. "The painful suture will seem to begin pulsating. This pulsating will continue for a matter of minutes. As the pulsation gradually subsides, so will the pain." (Osteopathic Annals, p. 30/241) It is interesting to note that this description was not brought to my attention until well after a similar method of palpations of various pulsations had been incorporated into B.E.S.T. on the cranium and other areas of the body as well.

B.E.S.T. functions on the premise that this "life-force" or nerve energy flows freely through a well-balanced body when the pulses throughout the body are synchronized. Conversely, interference in the transmission of nerve energy exists when pulses in different parts of the body are not synchronized.

Clinical experience has shown that communication with subconscious areas of the body can be established through contact with these pulses. Robert O. Becker, M.D., a leading researcher in the field of electromagnetic influence on the body, has stated, "Since all living things generate weak electromagnetic fields, and since many, if not all, can sense those of the earth, communication by this medium remains a strong possibility." (Becker and Selden, p. 166) When these pulses are synchronized, the body is in a state of homeostatic equilibrium.

Maintaining homeostasis can be equated with maintaining health. Richard Gerber, M.D., writes in his recent book *Vibrational Medicine: New Choices for Healing Ourselves:*

> From an energetic standpoint, the human body, when weakened or shifted from equilibrium, oscillates at a different and less harmonious frequency than when healthy. This abnormal frequency reflects a general state of cellular energetic imbalance within the physical body. When a weakened individual is unable to shift his/her energetic mode to the needed frequency (which allows their immune system to properly defend the body), a certain amount of subtle energetic help may be needed. If this same individual is supplied with a dose of the needed energetic frequency, it allows the cellular bioenergetic systems to resonate in the proper vibrational mode, thereby throwing off the toxicities of the illness. (Gerber, p. 210)

My clinical experience involving thousands of patients has shown that "subtle energetic help" can be administered through palpations by specific fingers of the doctor. The minute amount of energy transmitted through one individual to another exerts a dramatic influence on the patient's internal communication system.

The importance of "electrodynamic fields" is also addressed by Harold Saxon Burr, Ph.D. and former faculty member of the Yale University School of Medicine, in his book *Blueprint for Immortality*. It is this electromagnetic element that B.E.S.T. utilizes to detect and update memory patterns that continue to circumscribe physiology for conditions that are no longer present.

Light pressure applied with the fingers to specific anatomical areas including spinal and cranial sites allows the body to recognize more appropriate structural configurations than those that exist in a symptomatic patient. Light pressure adjustments provide sensory information that allow the body to recognize and assume more appropriate structural configuration which, in turn, allows for improved organ function as the infinite, internal, innate intelligence reestablishes homeostasis.

Tapping Into Universal Pulses

Palpating specific contact points on the patient's cranium and torso is a fundamental procedure of B.E.S.T. However, even more important than searching out the most appropriate contact points is the doctor's attitude toward the patient.

We have been discussing the effects electromagnetic fields have on all living systems. One of the most potent effectors of fields is the energy produced by thoughts. The energy of thoughts has a greater effect on the energy field of an individual than any other function of the body. Through thoughts we can facilitate or inhibit health. Patients themselves affect their health every minute of every day by their thought processes. And, the doctors the patients turn to for help in overcoming pain or illness affect their patients' health by their own thoughts.

Positive, non-judgmental thoughts by a doctor, accompanied by strong visualization on the part of the patient, react with the patients' individual fields to bring them more in tune with universal energy.

THE HEALING FIELD

12

What Others Say About... Physiologic Pulses

One of the first observations I made in the early developmental stages of B.E.S.T. was the presence of small subcutaneous nodules around the spinal region, presumably invisible to the naked eye yet easily detectable by palpation even through several layers of clothing. These nodules (to which I assigned the "technical" terminology "peas") consistently showed three attributes: (1) they were tender upon palpation, (2) they disappeared after a brief period of palpation, and (3) they pulsated. When two "peas" were palpated simultaneously, the pulsations could be felt to be first asynchronous, then synchronous. Of course, the first thought was that these were pulsations associated with the cardiovascular system. However, the pulses occurred in locations of the body other than those of arteries or veins, and they were not beating in unison. I found that when the pulsating "peas" were asynchronous, even slight pressure on them caused pain. However, when the pulsations became synchronous, both pain and "pea" subsided. Physiologic pulses play an important role in B.E.S.T. procedures.

Four definite motions have been observed at operation:
1. A pulsation which is synchronous with cardiac contractions.
2. A pulsation which coincides with respiratory pressure changes associated with inhalation and exhalation.

3. A wave not related to either heart rate or respiration but one which constantly maintains its own cycle.
4. An undulating pulsation which has not been identified. [Magoun, pp 23-24. 1976]

Hyden and others showed that glial cells, grown in tissue culture, pulsate continuously. [Magoun, p. 24. 1976]

The evidence now available suggests that all objects, and especially living objects, contain, are surrounded by, and interact with clouds of diffuse matter-energy at least some of which has been radiated to the earth from the sun. I describe these clouds as composed of diffuse relativistic superconducting plasma. Relativistic considerations lead to the conclusion that it is impossible for an *outside* observer to measure most physical parameters *inside* that plasma system. Nevertheless, the system can be expected to make its presence known by effects it produces on physical parameters *outside* itself, and these outside effects should be measurable by an *outside* observer. Such outside effects may be accentuated by applied high voltages, as in Kirlian photography, and may reveal themselves by synchronization of electromagnetic oscillations in adjacent molecules resulting in laser action with observable electromagnetic emissions. [Cope, 1980, p 350]

Hearts from 2 to 3-day-old rats were used for culturing by the procedure originally described by Harary and Farley (1963). . . . the hearts removed aseptically . . . then transferred to a sterile Petri dish . . . . The five individual heart cell harvests were then pooled together. . . . The cells were then plated in plastic disposable Petri dishes at a concentration of 5×10^6 cells per plate. The cultures were then incubated at 37°C with 5% CO_2 and 95% air. In 24 to 48 hr, the cells attach to the bottom of the Petri dishes and begin to contract. By 3 to 4 days after culturing, the cells are beating in unison at about 125 to 175 contractions per minute and are ready for study. [Miletich, *et al.*, p 182. 1983]

Extracellular electric fields oscillating in the range of EEG frequencies have been measured with microelectrodes (Elul, 1962, 1972) and have revealed a magnitude between 2 and 5 V/m. They appear to vary little with depth over vertical distances of the order of 1 mm. [Tourenne, p. 498. 1985]

The theory of long range coherence in biological systems proposed by Frohlich (1968, 1972) shows that the supply of energy above a threshold to a system of polar membrane proteins leads to a coherent electric oscillation between a strongly polar excited state and a weakly polar ground state. For frequencies in the range of 1 to 100 GHz, long range interactions along the "greater membrane " (Schmitt & Samson, 1970) bring large regions of that membrane to oscillate coherently. Frohlich has suggested that large regions of the cortex can also be synchronously active at very low frequency because of such long range electrical interactions at microwave frequencies (Frohlich, 1972). [Tourenne, p. 500. 1985]

We conclude that the hanging drop technique is a simple and very demonstrative proof of the presence of natural oscillating fields about living cells. [Rivera, *et al*, p 54. 1985]

Whenever two or more oscillators in the same field are pulsing at *nearly* the same time, they tend to 'lock in' so that they are pulsing at *exactly* the same time. The reason, simply stated, is that nature seeks the most efficient energy state, and it takes less energy to pulse in cooperation than in opposition. Entrainment is so ubiquitous, in fact, that, as with the air we breathe, we hardly notice it. Yet it offers dramatic witness of the tendency toward perfect rhythm that we discover whenever we examine the roots of our existence. [Leonard, p 13-14. 1986]

The simplest single-celled organism oscillates to a number of different frequencies, at the atomic, molecular, subcellular, and cellular levels.... [Leonard p 14-15. 1986]

Let us assume that a population of neurons is charging and firing at a certain rate, say a known brain rhythm. Noise, accounting, for example, for random cross talk among neurons, causes each neuron to randomly change phase during its firing. (Note that this can also be seen as a random-frequency firing.) The firings are in principle completely incoherent among the neurons. When a certain degree of coherence is randomly established we are more likely to observe oscillations in the spontaneous EEG or MEG, where a large number of neuron outputs are summed (alpha rhythm, for example). If a stimulation is applied, it would cause a similar phase change, but larger and time-correlated for the whole population of neurons. Under certain conditions the stimulus (say the first one) is able to phase-lock (or synchronise) some of the spontaneous firings, therefore increasing the degree of coherence. If the successive stimulus is in phase with the temporal behavior of the neuron, then a larger number of neurons would be synchronised, and so on, until saturation. It is apparent that only in the hypothesis of 'resonant' stimulation, could each successive stimulus synchronise other neurons. If the stimulation is out of resonance, successive stimuli would destroy previously established synchronisation. This model is consistent with the one suggested by Basar (1980) for a simpler case. [Barone, *et al.*, p 75. 1987]

... biological effects in animal and culture models ... confirm that PEMFs affected cellular processes pertinent to bone repair. [Bassett, p 36. 1987]

Several other reports indicate that PEMFs affect local mineralization processes but not total body calcium metabolism. [Bassett, p. 36. 1987]

Investigations have noted similarities in PEMF effects and the calcium-blocker action of Verapamil. [Bassett, p. 37. 1987]

How specific are the actions of PEMFs? Do changes in energy patterns result in different effects? Several examples have been cited already. A burst elevates calcium content, whilst a single pulse lowers it. [Bassett, p. 38. 1987]

... when a biological system is exposed to a given pulse it may respond in one manner if parallel to B, another at right angles to B, another in the central axis of B and yet another if peripherically located. [Bassett, p. 39. 1987]

Selected PEMFs improve the rate of peripheral nerve regeneration and function, promote growth of new small blood vessels (angio genesis) and modify the local action of certain hormones. [Bassett, p. 40. 1987]

Since almost every physiological and psychological correlate is manifested as an ultraradian rhythm, all having similar periodicities, Werntz et al. (1981) suggested that the hypothalamus was responsible for the regulation and integration of the various rhythmic phenomena. The hypothalamus is known to be the major control center for ANS function. This proposed organization presents a new inclusive and expansive view of the ANS-CNS relationship. [Srinivasan, p 100. 1988]

... minute electric currents, as small as a few millionths of an ampere or even less, are associated with heartbeat, brain electrical activity, eye movements, etc., and are in the frequency range of a fraction of a Hz to a few Hz. By the well-known principle of electromagnetic induction, they induce time-varying magnetic fields of the same frequency and strength as small as a few parts per million-million of a Tesla -pico-Tesla (pT) or even much smaller, femto-Tesla (fT). These unbelievably minute magnetic fields have, during the last few years, attracted the attention of the medical profession. [Srinivasan, p 187. 1988]

Experimental data also indicate the existence of *an energy anatomy and physiology*, the internal structure and function of organisms on energy dimensions. Not only do we recognize the transmission of information along the nerves by bioelectric pulses with a frequency spectrum extending to thousands of hertz, but we recognize EMF interactions occurring within the organism. Much remains to be discovered about internal energetic organization. With development of the SQUID (Superconducting Quantum Interference Device), magnetic measurement has been greatly assisted, permitting exploration of delicate EMF phenomena inside the organism that are not measurable with electrical means. [Srinivasan, pp 11, 13. 1988]

Highly coherent oscillations can act as carriers for modulation representing a control function for the regulation and maintainance of homeostasis in living systems. Certain groups of atoms called 'free radicals' are essential to the chemistry whereby oxygen- burning organisms generate their energy but they are capable of interacting strongly with electromagnetic fields as well as being highly reactive chemically. [Simon & Best, p 34. 1989]

The basis of the body's 'hard-wired' telecommunications network is the excitable nerve cell. This is stimulated to give its action potential by depolarising the cell membrane with a destabilising pulse which exceeds the thermal energy of 25mV. A current then flows externally to the cell; simultaneously, a net positive ion current flows into the cell through the membrane. This gives rise to a potential gradient around the cell which can be detected by external electrodes and can also trigger other excitable cells into producing their action-potential pulses. [Smith & Best, p 60. 1989]

The condition of the physical body is affected not only by the rate of etheric energy flow, but also by the degree of harmony in its rhythm, and any obstructions which deform the normal energy patterns result in loss of vitality and ill health. [Shafica, p 38. 1989]

The Healing Field

13

Reconnecting The Mind

"Memory is an active process, not a passive one; it changes, distorts, and adapts the remembered materials so that they will fit better into preconceived schemata."
— Hans Eysenck, English psychologist

Chiropractic, like medicine, traditionally focuses on the physical ills of its patients. Outside the fields of psychiatry and psychology, only cursory interest is aroused in the physician to the thoughts, beliefs, fears, and concerns of patients — to the "mind."

In our highly technological, scientifically-oriented world, we tend to see as health determinants only the physical and quantifiable: matter, substances, events, reactions that can be weighed, measured, or observed. The abstract, or non-quantifiable, is relegated to the realm of the supernatural, fantasy, speculation, or mysticism. A not-always-clear division separates the physical from the abstract. However, with our sophisticated instruments, more and more formerly "abstract" concepts can be regarded as "physical ." We have now devised equipment to harness energies and measure and monitor elements of nature that only a matter of decades ago were regarded as fantasies of science fiction writers. Men walking on the moon. Laser surgery. "Smart" bombs. Superconductors. The structure of DNA. SQUID. We are now able to measure smaller and smaller components of nature, and, in the process, are converting formerly abstract concepts into physical "reality."

History shows us that knowledge does not create reality. The earth has been round all along despite the "accepted" view that it was flat. Cells didn't come into being only when they were first viewed in the 17th century. The healing arts and sciences must be open to concepts of abstracts that relate to healing and health.

Despite modern technological accomplishments, we still have not been able to accurately identify or quantify that illusive entity scientists, philosophers, and laity alike acknowledge exist that is perhaps the greatest abstract of all: the mind. We can't describe the mind itself—only its effects: what it does. We talk about "losing one's mind," or "changing one's mind," or "keeping in mind," or "expanding his mind," or "being of two minds." Yet we still can't pinpoint where or what that mind is. Despite these deficiencies in quantification, we know the "mind" exists. Philosophers and thinkers have pondered whether the mind is a material or immaterial entity for over 2500 years.

Of the lengthy descriptions given in *Webster's Third New International Dictionary, Unabridged*, one best describes the faculty and the focus of the concepts discussed in this book: "mind . . . the conscious element or factor in the universe that in dualistic metaphysical systems is contrasted with matter and in monistic idealistic systems is held to be the only ultimate reality: spirit, nous, intelligence."

This dichotomy of thought (of the mind) is the crux of the concepts put forth in this book: the dualistic nature of man (mind and body are separate entities inhabiting a common structure) or the monositic nature of man (mind and body are an interwoven unit that makes man distinctively "man"). Other than the small segments of medicine of psychiatry or psychology, and despite research and admonitions by some of its peers to the contrary, conventional modern science functions in under an unspoken dualistic premise: disease is exclusively a "body" function. Identify and treat the offending organ or system of the body and the problem is solved.

In recent years, volumes have been written by highly educated scientists and laymen to illustrate that the mind—how a person thinks—affects that person's physical well-being. In addition, more volumes have been written describing how thoughts and attitudes affect an individual's success in business, relationships, society, and life in general. Yet few (if any) explain why. By understanding that mental activity generates energy, and that this energy is transferred into the energy fields of the body, we can understand why thoughts and the mind are so important in gaining, restoring, or maintaining physical health. And, in keeping with our conviction that the mind and body are inextricably related, we can see that thoughts affect the physiology of the body.

Surviving To Defend While Defending To Survive

Man individually and mankind corporately are designed to survive. The primary function, initiated subconsciously, of every physiological process and reaction (including thinking) is to survive the moment. Man was not designed specifically to be comfortable while he is surviving. Comfortable, pain-free survival is a goal of individuals; however, comfort is not necessary for survival. Regardless of the comfort level produced by any physiological activity, all functions of the body are directed toward the entity maintaining life at that precise instant.

In order to survive, we must defend against conditions and elements that threaten that survival. In our society, those conditions and elements of everyday living that must be defended against are as diverse as improper food, air pollution, hazards of traffic, perhaps, even, physical assault, and countless other by-products of modern society.

Catalysts for defense come in many forms. A dramatic illustration of a defense-producing physical event would be falling off a ladder. Without thought, arms and legs flail in an effort to abort the fall, muscles tense, adrenalin flows. A less dramatic but equally as potent stimulus of defense is the sudden appearance in the car's rear-view mirror of a flashing blue light accompanied by the distinctive wail of a police-car siren. Instantly, the same physiological responses as those generated by more physical threats occur: muscles tense, digestion subsides, pupils dilate, adrenalin flows. Yet the blue-light situation is entirely different from the falling situation. There is no immediate threat to life and limb. Nonetheless, the response of the body is the same: defense physiology brought about by the adrenal response.

Defense physiology is literally a life-saver. Without these autonomic responses, we would have to consciously evaluate each situation and determine what if any action was needed. In the short time all of this thinking and deciding takes, the opportunity for an effective defense response would probably have passed and disaster a *fait accompli*.

Defense physiology is a physiologic response activated by the subconscious in response to sensorially perceived external stimuli *or to internal stimuli of thoughts accompanied by feelings*. Little physiological response accompanies unexciting mental activity such as reading a junk-mail flyer touting a sale at the local bird feed outlet; however, a great deal of physiological response usually accompanies noticing, opening, and reading a notice of impending audit from the IRS, or a court summons, or an eviction notice. The actions for perceiving both junk-mail and an IRS notice are the same: the reactions are entirely different. The difference is in the mental interpretations of the perceptions.

Most defense physiology in our society is brought about by internal, non-physical threats: emotions. Anger, worry, prolonged fear, jealousy, hurt, grief, and all of the other emotions we term "negative" bring about defense physiology. Defense brought about by negative emotions can be devastating to the body and to health. Defense brought about by actual external emergencies — accidents, physical attacks, alerts of impending disaster and the like — is natural, normal, and necessary. The difference between internal emotionally-induced defense physiology and external emergency-induced defense physiology is that the external emergency situation ends relatively quickly, and the body can return to its natural homeostatic function. Internal emotionally-induced defense physiology, however, often has no discernable end. Situations that foster the defense go on and on, and even after the situation ends, the memory, consciously or subconsciously, lingers.

Defense physiology generated by thoughts and attitudes is ordinarily more potent, therefore more detrimental to health. Thoughts and attitudes are accompanied by feelings. Strong feelings (negative feelings more so than positive feelings) are cemented in memory along with the memory of the event that triggered the feelings. In fact, my clinical experience shows that the suppressed memory of the feelings can outlive the conscious memory of the event that precipitated the feelings.

Nearly every patient who consults a health care specialist of any discipline is functioning under emotionally-induced defense physiology. The body is, and has been, defending against a perceived threat. The body was designed to prepare itself for defense. However, it was not designed to withstand days, weeks, months, or years of unremitting defense without damage. In time, the body becomes exhausted. The body cannot defend and replenish at the same time. As a result, the immune system suffers, and the maintenance and repair functions are suppressed. The stage is set for disease, and symptoms begin to become evident.

Treating symptoms brought on by continuous defense physiology is futile. If one symptom is suppressed, another will appear. Eliminating symptoms may increase the comfort level of the patient for a while, but it won't correct the cause that brought on the symptoms. The cause of defense, and, consequently, the ultimate cause of pain and disease brought on by sustained defense physiology, is in the patient's thoughts.

For years, the verdict of doctors encountering symptoms for which they could find no discernable physical cause has been that the patient was suffering from psychosomatic illness: "it's all in your mind." We can see that not only are allegedly psychosomatic complaints products of the mind, but symptoms, with sources verified by examination or laboratory tests, stem from "the patient's mind." The way a patient thinks governs the way his body functions. If the patient worries constantly, or fears losing his job, or hates his father, or is jealous of others, or lives in an ongoing financial crisis, or is constantly under negative stress of any kind, that patient will eventually become sick. Prolonged defense physiology mandates illness.

Self Esteem And Self Disdain

One of the greatest, if not *the* greatest, conscious determinant of health is the patient's attitude toward himself. Outward displays of bravado, confidence, egocentricity, or self-assurance frequently mask inward convictions of self-inadequacy, ineptness, stupidity, victimhood, unattractiveness, or even self-disgust. No matter how convincing an outward show of favorable self-esteem a patient may put on, if the inner conviction is that of self-disdain, the body responds defensively — it defends against a multitude of perceived threats and negativity.

Self-esteem and self-disdain are the products of accumulated thoughts and beliefs; the responses self-esteem or self-disdain induce in the body are the products of feelings. Lives there a man whose life has been so pristine that he has not committed a minor social or business gaff, or been ridiculed by a boss, parent, or other "significant other"? Minor indiscretions or public ridicule generate feelings of embarrassment, shame, or humiliation to the very core of the sufferer's being. These feelings are often relived when the incident is recalled. It is feelings that produce physiological responses of blushing, sweating, nervous activity, and defense, and the pattern of the response to the feelings (defense) is embedded in memory along with the memory of the event itself. When the incident is recalled, or when an another incident occurs to bring about similar feelings, the pattern of response that has already been established sets in motion the same physiological activity. Memory recalls more than just pictures; memory colors self-esteem.

Accrued feelings about oneself dictate the level of self-esteem. If the patient feels good about himself, his body is allowed to function normally and naturally without defending itself; both his self-esteem and health flourish. If he dislikes himself, for whatever reason, his body is continually defensive, functions in a survival mode; both his health and self-esteem suffer.

Mind, Thoughts, And The Universal Energy

Perhaps you have questioned why some people breeze through life with few major catastrophes, good health, success at just about everything they try, and a generally good attitude. Doctors don't see many of these people on a regular basis, just for emergencies or routine checkups. Are these "have it all" people happy, enthusiastic, full of vitality and satisfied with their lot because they are healthy, successful and think well of themselves? Or, are they healthy, successful and think well of themselves because they are happy, enthusiastic, full of vitality, and satisfied?

Reconnecting The Mind

My clinical experience shows that the latter is true. Those whose thought processes, beliefs, and attitudes (1) focus on the best possible outcomes, and (2) are judiciously oblivious to the prospect of "bad luck" or disaster are the "winners" in life.

The flip side of that coin shows the same pattern. Those who view life as a tumultuous stream of crises, "bad luck," disasters, broken relationships, lost jobs, financial crises, and declining health are, in the main, conforming to those views. Those whose thoughts, beliefs and attitudes accept and expect that "if it can go wrong, it will," are seldom disappointed.

How does this happen?

The first explanation, as can be heard from just about any motivational lecturer, is that when we have a goal firmly in mind , we subconsciously work to reach that goal. No matter whether the outcome we expect and subconsciously work toward is positive or negative, our beliefs and attitudes program our subconscious to reach the destination or goal we have set. "I knew I was going to spill that drink." "I knew I wasn't going to get that job." When we convince ourselves that a given outcome will occur, if we have anything to do with it, most of the time our projections will be realized.

Each of us reaches his own level of subconscious expectations. But, there is more to it than conscious/subconscious programming.

We point out in this book that each of us has his own energy field that envelops us and interacts with other energy fields. All energy fields contain all information, just as the DNA in one cell of the body contains the same information as the DNA is all other cells of the body. Energy information is transmitted from the field to the body, and from the body to the field. The body/mind is both a receiver and a transmitter. When the energy frequencies of the mind are synchronized with the energy frequencies of the fields, field/mind homeostasis is the result. When the energy of the fields outside the visible body (the universal energy fields) and the energy of the body/mind resonate harmoniously, health, success, and happiness result. When the energy fields are not resonating harmoniously, disease, pain, or even death is the product.

Dynamic, Vibrating Energy

The common goal of the doctor and patient is to help the patient restructure his thoughts and beliefs to establish a resonance with health.

Thoughts govern a patient's life. Positive thoughts, negative thoughts, happy thoughts, sad thoughts, all reverberate through the physical system we call the body. Yet the impact of thoughts isn't contained within the skin. Energy of thoughts radiates from within to the field that surrounds the body. We know that energy flows from the body. Electroencephalograms record on the outside of the body energy emitted from the brain. Electrocardiograms record on the outside of the body energy emitted from the heart muscle.

Electromagnetic activity within the body radiates from the body. The body, then, is more than the physical entity visible to the naked eye. It is made up of more than the physical entities viewed under an electronmicroscope or through x-ray film. The body is more than the sum of its parts, and that "more" is the electromagnetic field which radiates beyond the material bones, muscles, internal organs and skin.

Yet, the system is even more complex than that. The energy doesn't just dissipate aimlessly into the air. It constitutes a dynamic field around the body. The body field does not exist in isolation any more than does the body itself. The field of the body connects and mingles with the earth's fields and the fields of other nearby living systems. We are connected through these interwoven fields to the fields of every other being, creature, and object. More than that, we are connected directly to the universe itself, and the vitality and resonance of each individual's field contributes or detracts from contiguous or interrelated fields.

Energy and information are constantly exchanged among interconnecting fields. Just as radio waves, electric lines and the vast armada of electrical and electronic equipment that saturates our country contribute to the electromagnetic fields in which we live, energy from individuals is a part of the overall electromagnetic complex.

Energy comes in a variety of forms: light, heat, electricity, gravity, magnetism, sound. And each of these forms resonates at a different rate. Just as a submicroscopic system changes when it gives off or absorbs a discrete amount of energy, we can assume that larger systems also change when energy is emitted or received.

The hypotheses presented in this book are based on the premise that vibrating energies are common to the universe, the earth, and all systems and entities. Primary power (prime mover) of these energies permeates the universe and all that is in it. This field of primary energy is behind all creation and is perfect to keep the universe and all of its components in balance. Equilibrium with this primary source is reached when the energies of lesser or smaller systems resonate with the primary energy. Energy fields of each system in the universe interact in the fashion of concentric circles with proximate fields, which in turn react with the ultimate field. The universe, with its diverse energy fields, functions as a unit, just as the body with its diverse systems functions as a unit. When one field is affected, the effect resounds throughout the system.

Since the mind harbors and develops thoughts, and the thoughts themselves all radiate energy from the body to the surrounding fields, the way we think controls not only the physiology of the body but also the vitality of the external energy field.

An Encyclopaedia Britannica contributor wrote in a short section entitled "Some Speculations on Energy": "The concept of energy has demonstrated a remarkable survivability in the rapidly expanding understanding of the nature of things. To a large extent this survivability is no doubt a result of its adaptability to cover an increasingly complex set of phenomena that are revealed as ability to observe the physical world increases. . . . Indeed, it would appear that the concept of energy has value not only in explaining the readily observable physical world but, when data accumulate that cannot be explained with the incomplete facts, the use of the concept of the conservation of energy can be very helpful in indicating where to look for missing answers. . . . Perhaps the data that have been collected have been obtained by observing quantities on only one-half of the universe." (Britannica, 18:447 2b) Or, to put it another way, perhaps we have been viewing our

The Healing Field

world, including the factors that determine health, from the wrong angle.

We believe only what we understand. And, we don't understand something until it is familiar to us. Until we have acquired experience or thoughts that can reflect what we see, we have trouble absorbing new information. We have to have a basis for interpreting what we observe. When our observations conflict with what we already "know," these observations may not register. In the world of health, we "understand" and are comfortable with the chemical/mechanical model. Consequently, we may have trouble "seeing" a less tangible model. The anecdote recounted in the book *Energy Medicine* gives us food for thought that can be applied to how we see the mind-body continuum:

> Let us remember that our models also shape and limit our perceptions. When Charles Darwin anchored his ship, Beagle, off the coast of the island of Patagonia, he sent a landing party ashore in small rowboats. Amazingly, the Patagonian natives watching from shore were blind to the Beagle, but easily saw the rowboats. They had no prior experience of sailing ships, but were familiar with canoes. Rowboats, which were similar to canoes, fit their model of the world, but the brigantine did not. [Srinivasan, p. 20]

14

Intentional Healing

Resonating With Health

Resonance is the key to health. The resonance of the body responding to the frequency of its personal surrounding field. Burr indicates that the field is the template for the body. The field sets the tone of the body. If the frequency (or rhythm) of the field is not synchronized with the frequency of the primary energy source of the universe, the body will also be out of synch.

The body resonates with its contiguous field. Resonate: vibrate sympathetically (as with some source of sound or electric oscillations). [*Webster's Third New International Dictionary, Unabridged,* 1986]

If the body is a "reflection" of its field, and if the frequency of the field is not quite synchronized with the universal field, then the body does not resonate with the universal field: pain, illness, depression, disease must occur.

What determines the frequency of the patient's field? And, how can the doctor, or the patient, "re-tune" the field to reduce pain or bring about health?

The primary "nurturer" of the "self-field" is thoughts. For most people, most of the time, those affecting thoughts are self-generated. Energy of each thought that is accompanied by feelings "feeds" the self-field. When the thoughts and feelings are positive — love, joy, forgiveness, contentment — the self-field is fed with positive energy. On the other hand, when the self-field is fed with negative energy — fear, hate, judgment, bigotry, jealousy, anxiety, and all of the other emotions that "ruin your day" — the field is diminished.

Positive energy adds to the field: it "feeds" the field and is field-enhancing. Negative energy diminishes the field: it negates (or neutralizes the positive energy of) the field and is field-destroying.

The thoughts of the patient determine the "health" of the field, and the "health" of the field determines the physical (and mental) health of the patient.

The next most important factor that determines the health of the self-field is the substances that go into the patient's body. Food, drugs (either prescription, over-the counter, or recreational, including alcohol and nicotine), atmospheric pollutants, electromagnetic pollution of man-made equipment, or other substances. Food is first on this list because everyone consumes food. Not everyone uses drugs, lives in a highly polluted city or agricultural area, or lives under high-tension power lines. Everyone eats. The type of food the patient eats affects the energy of his self-field. Highly-processed foods are particularly field-destructive. Microwaved foods, of which the molecular structure has been altered, teeters between neutral and negative. However, the negative effects of inappropriate food can be greatly diminished by feeding the field the positive energy of field-enhancing thoughts.

Most people come into this world resonating harmoniously with the perfect primary power of the universe. As infants, they receive positive energy from loving parents. Infants are oblivious to negativity around them. They give and receive unconditional love. Only the most hard-hearted cynic (uncomprisingly negative, through and through) can resist the vibrant, outflowing nonjudgmental smile of a tiny child untainted by negative experiences of life.

A newborn (ideally) comes into this world as a part of a loving family. The infant can do nothing except be. Yet, his mother and father exude love toward him. He doesn't earn love. It is given to him unconditionally. His first experiences in life are manifestations of his mother's and father's attitude that he, the child, is perfect. Initially, the infant knows nothing other than the perfection of this perfect love.

Then, as the parents respond to the day-to-day care of the child, they experience minor or major inconveniences: the child cries; he sleeps all day and is awake all night; he has trouble keeping his food down; he requires constant attention. As these incidents pile one on top of the other, the mother and/

or father begins to experience frustration. Positive unconditional love is still there. However, the negativity of frustration, annoyance, or, perhaps, downright hostility on the part of the parents overrides the positive on many occasions. The child experiences new feelings that are contrary to the feelings brought about by receiving unconditional love.

As the child experiences the vagaries of life, either first hand or through his parents, these experiences are recorded in his memory. The feelings that accompany the experiences are also recorded. Although the child cannot verbalize his feelings, nonetheless, feelings exist. And, although memories of infancy and toddlerhood are, for the most part, irretrievable to the person as adults, the impressions of the memories remain fixed. And, additional memories and feelings are generated every day of the child's life: memorable experiences of childhood and adolescence aren't noted for positiveness. Consequently, most people reach adulthood already thoroughly contaminated by negative thoughts, negative feelings, negative beliefs, and habits of attitude that perpetuate them; habits that assure that the self-field will receive negative energy thereby diminishing the vibrancy of the field and of the energy projected back to the body.

The body is a reflection of the self-field. The body resonates with the field. When the resonance of the field is distorted, the energy reflected back to the body is distorted.

Tuning The Field

Only the patient can heal himself. Only the patient can control his thoughts. And, only the patient's conscious and subconscious thoughts and feelings direct his physiology.

Drugs, surgery, chiropractic adjustments, acupuncture, and other attempts to promote healing can interrupt conscious and subconscious thought-generated, autonomic physiological functions. Externally imposed stimuli can, and do, alter the way the body functions. The stronger the stimuli (drugs or adjustments) the greater the effect on entities and processes within the body. When individual entities or responses of the body are affected through medications, adjustments or surgery, the system of which that entity or response is an integral part is affected which in turn affects other systems and functions of the body. For example, anti-inflammatory drugs to relieve inflammation and pain of arthritis patients. Prolonged use of anti-inflammatories that mimic the body's cortisol affects more than inflamed joints. Guyton writes: "... administration of large doses of cortisol causes significant atrophy of all the lymphoid tissue throughout the body, which in turn decreases the output of both T cells and antibodies from the lymphoid tissue. As a result, the level of immunity for almost all foreign invaders of the body is decreased." (Guyton, p 917.) We call these unintentional alterations of the body's function "side effects."

Some patients and medical doctors consider side effects to be tolerable as long as the primary purpose is achieved. In the example of the arthritic who is looking for immediate relief from ongoing pain, the prospect of greater susceptibility to other diseases down the road is a fair trade-off. If we accept that it was the patient's thoughts over the years that reduced the resonance of his self-field, we can see that the body was forced to respond to an internally-generated threat. We can also see that by addressing the patient's attitudes and thoughts and eliminating the internal threat, the resonance of the self-field will be restored, the body will reflect the health of the field, and the body will function naturally, the way it was designed — without arthritis.

Every time an external influence is imposed on the body, the whole body is affected. Some element, organ, or system of the body responds by either increasing activity or decreasing activity. When these alterations occur, the body's inner intelligence signals compensatory changes in other parts of the body. Although the symptom being treated may improve, the compensations the body must make to externally induced interference may prove too much for the survival mechanisms to handle. And the interference transmitted to the self-field may be of such magnitude as to destroy the positive components of the already depleted energy field. The warped adage "the operation was a success, but the patient died" exemplifies the extremes of externally induced side effects.

Content And Intent

Potential doctors are selected from the cream of the educational system. They are trained to use their intelligence to analyze symptoms, select a course of treatment, and administer specific therapies or rituals. Yet the foundation of healing is not in the content of the cerebral cortex but in the intent of the doctor's inner wisdom. Inner wisdom and intent do not come from books, labs, clinics, or rounds. Intent comes from attitude. From the internal "mind" as opposed to the intellectual mind.

Every ministration of every health-care professional is directed by the conscious mind, the brain, the intellect of the doctor. The doctor responds to a patient's specific complaints according to education and experience. Treatments and therapies are cortically inspired. Sometimes they work, sometimes they don't. Sometimes surgery helps a patient feel better (after the rigors of the surgery itself are over); sometimes it doesn't. Sometimes chiropractic adjustments work, sometimes they don't. The effectiveness of any therapeutic discipline doesn't depend entirely on the skill of a well-trained doctor; effectiveness depends on the *intent* of both the patient and the doctor.

Intention is a common ingredient in all types of healing, including chiropractic. When a patient consults a doctor of any discipline, the patient has a degree of confidence in that doctor. The patient intends to be better as a result of the doctor's treatment. By the same token, the doctor has been educated and trained to believe in the type of work he or she does. The doctor *intends* for the patient to be better as a result of treatment.

Without positive intention on the part of the patient, healing is impeded. Also without positive intention on the part of the doctor, healing may occur, but that effect is despite the doctor's efforts, not a result. Doctors who have lost confidence in the therapies they administer, even if they are expert technicians in their field, become less effective as healers. Without confidence in their technique, their intention to heal falters. And the reverse is also true. Doctors who may lack the degree of technical expertise enjoyed by some of their peers are often more successful than their more highly trained colleagues because they are intent upon helping their patients. Intent of the doctor can be more effective than content of the doctor's brain.

Intent is not to be confused with wishful thinking. Intent is a dynamic force that comes from within the body. Intent is not dependent upon the content of the cerebral cortex. Wishful thinking is a superficial "wouldn't it be nice" passing thought. Wishful thinking, by definition, is wishing for something that reason and rationality cortically judge to be impossible.

Positive intention on the part of the doctor influences the patient's self-field. The patient may be so sick that both his intention and energy field are weak. However, the doctor who has the best interest of the patient at heart can project positive energy into the patient's waning field to boost the resonance of the field to a more healthful level.

A patient who has confidence in his doctor and is hopeful of a cure is receptive to the doctor's projected positive thoughts and energy. The doctor can reinforce this hope with reassurances such as, "I can help you." These reassurances not only increase the patient's level of hope (a positive thought and feeling), but the doctor's positiveness projects positive energy into the patient's field. With a receptive patient and a confident, positive doctor, the doctor serves as an amplifier of the perfect, positive, primary field to update the patient's self-field. The doctor's energy is projected into the patient's field and updates the resonance of that field. As the resonance improves, the patient improves. And as the resonance improves due to the doctor's intent, the patient's thoughts and attitudes become more positive, and the field resonance improves even more. As the patient's field resonance improves, his internal resonance improves because the field is a template for the body.

Negative Intent

People don't go to a doctor believing that the doctor is going to try to keep them sick. They go because they intend for the doctor to help them. They have hope. And, hope is a highly positive force.

The greatest factor in healing is intent. Intent of the doctor, and intent of the patient. But suppose the doctor has lost confidence in specific procedures customarily used in specific instances. Like the doctor who tells a patient, "This is how we are going to treat your problem, but I must tell you, it probably won't help"; or, "we'll try this, but if it doesn't work, we'll try something else." What is the intent in these situations? What is intended when a doctor undertakes a particular course of therapy that, as far as the doctor is concerned, has a poor track record of healing?

A doctor who believes, whether that belief is expressed to the patient or not, that the therapy being administered is ineffective is practicing with *negative intent*. In the process, the doctor is projecting a negative force to the patient's already impaired field. However, despite these negative projections, the patient may improve. The hope and positiveness most patients take with them when they seek a doctor's help overrides the negative intent of the doctor.

Most doctors would vehemently deny ever having negative intent toward either their healing methods or their patients. Yet, negative intent is a product of cortical medicine. Modern medicine relies primarily on drugs and surgery to bring about changes in symptoms. Both drugs and surgery force the body to respond to emergency situations. Every drug in the body must be processed, detoxified, and eliminated. The body must defend against such intrusions. However, we know that drugs often relieve symptoms — at least temporarily. If drugs are a negative force causing the body to defend itself, why are drugs effective?

The administration of drugs carries along with it implied hope. The implication is that the drugs will bring about a positive change. This hope is positive energy. When the hope is shared by both the doctor and the patient, more positive energy is projected into the patient's field. This is why patients experience a positive response from the negative force of drugs. Two factors are involved: stimulation, caused by processing the drugs as they are being eliminated which causes symptomatology to change; and positive intent.

Most medical practitioners have faith, confidence and belief in the tools of their trade — drugs. They believe that they, through the content of their cortical intelligence, are directing the body to function differently. They assume that since the patient's body is malfunctioning that the body is inherently stupid and needs to be controlled from the outside. Yet they also know that not all patients respond favorably to treatment. They also know that malpractice is astronomically priced and that litigation has become almost commonplace. As a result, even doctors who have ultimate faith in their abilities to help people may experience negative intent. They must, for self-preservation, entertain the thought that the patient may not improve, and they must caution the patient that the treatment may not be effective. They must, because of experience and societal pressure, practice defensive intent. This attitude is detrimental both to the doctor and the patient. The doctor is less effective, and the patient comes away with dashed — or, at least, reduced — hope. When the hope, or positive intent, of the patient is impaired, healing is impaired.

Chiropractic has the advantage of depending on the positive, creative, healing force within the patient to restore health. Chiropractors are more prone to approach patients with positive intent. The chiropractic doctor knows that the patient's body is a self-healing, self-regulating, creative entity. As a result, the chiropractor is more able to approach each and every patient with positive intent: positiveness in the effectiveness of the technique being used and in the capabilities of the body. With this attitude, both the doctor and the patient respond favorably. The patient is given hope, and positive energy is directed to the patient's energy field through the positive thoughts and convictions of the chiropractor. The patient's field is fed a double dose of positiveness — his own, and that of the doctor.

Chiropractors who find their patients drifting away and their practices declining are usually suffering from practicing with negative, or indifferent intent. They have come to question the effectiveness of their technique, or they have begun to view their patients as "cases." Either way, their intent dwindled before their patient load.

Every practitioner of the healing arts — medicine man, witch doctor, neurosurgeon, chiropractor, internist, osteopath, . . . — projects energy to patients. This energy is positive or negative. It is impossible for a doctor dealing with patients not to project energy. Even "burnt out," tired, frustrated doctors, or those suffering from mental inertia, project energy to their patients. The doctor has some feeling toward patients, and that feeling carries with it energy that contributes or detracts from both the patient's energy field and the doctor's. The attitude and intent of medical doctors is generally determined by the faith they have in drugs. The attitude and intent of chiropractors is generally in the body's ability to heal itself. And intent is the most enduring medicine of all.

Intent, Double Blind Studies, And The Placebo Effect

Modern scientific investigators go to great lengths to assure that their procedures are completely unbiased and valid. The double-blind technique is considered to offer comparisons of products or therapies uncorrupted by personal biases or favoritism. Neither the subject nor the investigator knows whether the treatment the subject is receiving is designed to alter a condition of the subject or is merely an inert "look alike." Only at the conclusion of the study and analysis of the results is it known which data were the results of which treatment. Often, the subject never knows whether the treatment he received was the treatment being tested or the "placebo."

The word "placebo" comes from Latin, meaning "I shall please." Considering the premise that "intention" is a prime mover in healing, we can see that a placebo given in a double-blind study has a better than average chance of positively affecting the patient.

A conscientious, caring doctor who administers a therapy to a patient does so with the intent of helping that patient. There fore, no matter which therapy is used, as long as the doctor has confidence in it, that therapy will be beneficial. Results of double-blind studies rarely show that 100% of those treated with the active ingredient improved and that 100% of those receiving the placebo did not improve. Some patients in both camps improved, some in both did not improve. What causes this discrepancy? Perhaps there were more variations of physiological conditions than the investigators had realized among those who received the active therapy to keep some of them from benefitting. Perhaps those who benefitted from the placebo had been misdiagnosed. Then again, perhaps the difference in both groups was the intent of the administrator of the therapy.

If the administrator/doctor is aware that the study is being conducted, he or she will, with each prescription, experience a degree of suspicion as to whether this particular patient is receiving "real" therapy. This suspicion can be just enough to override the doctor's intention of healing. In the same manner, should the patient be aware he or she is involved in a test, the same suspicion or, worse, fear will be present. When fear intrudes, healing is hampered.

Now, if the administrator/doctor is not aware that the patient might be receiving spurious treatment, the doctor is as intent upon healing as ever. No suspicion or hesitancy clouds his intent. Even if the patient receives a placebo, intent — both the doctor's and the patient's — goes to work on the patient's external field to effect healing. The doctor puts positive "good" into the patient's field through positive intent. The patient improves under intentional healing.

The dispensation of placebos is not limited to double-blind studies. Some doctors will administer a placebo to a patient whose symptoms cannot be traced to a biological cause, or to a patient who uses complaints of imagined or minor aches and pains to the doctor as much needed social contact. In either instance, the patient often feels better and attributes the improvement to the doctor and the treatment. In these instances, although the doctor had neither faith nor confidence in the treatment, the patient had enough for both of them. The patient intended to get better.

So, we can see that, in reality, there is no such thing as a truly valid double-blind study, and there is no such thing as a placebo.

The value of therapies of any kind lie not in the content of the doctor's educated intelligence but in the intent of the doctor. A doctor who intends nothing but improvement for his or her patients is practicing intentional healing.

Intent. Does the doctor *intend* his or her therapies to work? Does the doctor *intend* his patient to get better? Intention is the common denominator of healing.

Intentional Healing

Chiropractic offers a vast scope of techniques. Some exert very little pressure. Some exert a great amount of pressure. Yet, all of them succeed most of the time. And, all of them fail sometimes. The technique isn't the only deciding factor. It's the intention. Every successful doctor believes that what he or she is doing is for the benefit of that patient. The doctor who ministers to people is successful. The doctor who treats "cases," is a technician.

Chiropractors have at least two important advantages in promoting healing: confidence that their adjustive techniques (whether forceful or non-forceful) will restore the natural healing properties of the body, and an unwavering belief that the body is a self-regulating, self-organizing, self-healing system from the inside out, above down, controlled by an innate force. Considering these and the many other advantages chiropractors bring to the healing arts, it becomes obvious why chiropractic has the potential of becoming the primary health care system of the twenty-first century as chiropractors work with positive intent as healing occurs.

Intent is a very important key to healing.

15

Working With The Healing Field

We have touched on the history of healing that set the stage for modern techniques. We reviewed briefly the trends that have directed man in his search to explain his condition. We have seen how man moved from the crediting forces in broad etherial world with dominion over health and disease, to investigations of the most minute units of the body to discover where things go wrong. In the early stages of the development of civilized man, before he discovered internal organs, the body was considered a complete entity, working in nature. Working only with those things discernable to his senses, and attributing to spirits or other "unseeables" those things he couldn't explain, man acknowledged his vulnerability to nature and his surroundings. The job of placating spirits to ward off disease or disaster was left to the medicine man, the conjurer, the priest, or the shaman.

Man acknowledged that there were powerful forces outside himself over which he had no control that influenced his entire life, and he played to those ubiquitous, sometimes vengeful, forces. Sacrifices, incantations, or whatever it took to ward off evil spirits and court the good. He believed in what he was doing and he met with a certain degree of success.

Yet, man is a creature of insatiable curiosity. He looks to explain the happenings in his life. If the reason he is sick is not obvious, he will attribute his condition to forces outside himself. If his experience denies to these explanations, he will continue to search for answers. Over time, in the civilized world, some of the more daring questioners discovered internal conditions that could account for ways the body functioned. With knowledge came a change of view. The further learned investigators

THE HEALING FIELD

delved into the inner workings of the body, the less attention was paid to the overall external influences on health and happiness.

Man has come a long way since the days of ignorance and superstition. However, we are now seeing signs that as far as health care is concerned, modern man may have thrown out the proverbial baby with the proverbial bathwater. By focusing on chemical reactions, neurons, hormones, DNA, and the thousands of other components we know of that make up the substantive mass of the body, we have lost sight, not only of the external influences that surround the body but also of the quality (or force) that constitutes "aliveness."

Centuries ago, man investigated "spirituality" or "religion" to understand the nature of his daily existence. In modern times, man investigates the physical to understand the nature of his daily existence. We, as a species, have gone from trying to understand the "big picture" to scrutinizing and disecting smaller and smaller parts of the whole in an effort to uncover the secrets of the body's minutiae. We have moved from a deductive form of study to an inductive form.

Yet, in the process of investigating smaller and smaller components of the physical, man is scientifically uncovering more and more abstractions, or "unexplainables." Scientific text books and papers offer conclusions of valid studies that state outright or imply that explanations for a given result cannot be explained. A case in point of "surprising findings" is the study reported in the highly esteemed British publication *Nature* of unexplainable reactions brought about by highly dilute solutions in which researchers "detected significant basophil degranulation down to the 1×10^{130} dilution." (p. 817) Publication of these findings caused quite a stir in the "scientific community" and elicited the following the caveat in an accompanying article in *Nature*:

> Benveniste's observations, on the other hand, are startling not merely because they point to a novel phenomenon, but because they strike at the roots of two centuries of observation and rationalization of physical phenomena. Where, for example, would elementary principles such as the Law of Mass Action be

if Benveniste is proved correct? The principle of restraint which applies is simply that, when an unexpected observation requires that a substantial part of our intellectual heritage should be thrown away, it is prudent to ask more carefully than usual whether the observation may be correct. (p. 787)

The premises, concepts, and ideas set forth in this book (and in all of my publications) are offered as summaries of analyses of my clinical findings, and the conclusions that have sprung from these findings. They are offered as grist for the investigative mill of others to confirm, elaborate, or refute.

The references quoted in this book are from a variety of books, articles, and papers written by well-credentialed investigators. The references are offered to illustrate that the tenets set forth in this book and my other writings fit with findings already published. The premises and practices of B.E.S.T. were not developed after searching the literature to find what might work. B.E.S.T. has developed — and continues to develop — through practical application of bits and pieces of knowledge gleaned through acknowledging and "listening" to the same universal intelligence credited in these pages with being the fountain of all knowledge, health, success and happiness.

My mission is to search for "truth" as a means to improve the health of mankind. Nothing in this book is considered the "final word"; we all are in a process of growing, learning, and expanding our intellectual horizons. However, I am firmly convinced by clinical success with actual patients that these concepts provide a basis for improving healing.

My ultimate goal as a doctor is to understand and to remove *primary* interference. In order to do this, I must be able to identify the primary force. I believe that all science has studied the *effects* of the same primary force I am looking for. And, I believe that, ultimately, that primary force will be found to be magnetism. I believe that magnetism is the primary force, and that gravity, heat, light, and electricity are all effects of magnetism in action. I believe that magnetism *is* the force that set our world, and universe, in motion billions of years ago. And I believe that our universe continues to be in the process of creating, second by second by second. However, with our limited concepts, we observe chaos and destruction at an equal rate.

The earth that appears stable to us moving about on it, is a living, dynamic, changing creation, constantly on the move. Along with its motion of rotation on its axis and around the sun, the magnetic fields are in a continuous state of change. Changes follow rhythmic patterns of eras, seasons, tides, and for stationary man, years, months, and days. Less obvious are changes in polarity.

Clear evidence exists indicating that polarity of the earth has switched several times in the course of its existence. Becker tells us that this reversal happens very quickly in geologic terms; not so quickly in terms of man. "All told, the change takes about five thousand years." [Becker and Selden, p 261] These polar switches may be viewed as evidence of a primary pulse of the earth and the universe.

We know that electromagnetic fields exist in and around the earth. We are beginning to understand that these fields are of substance. We can measure these field substances in terms of gauss and Hertz, yet we can't isolate them, pick them up and examine them. Nonetheless, we know they exist. The only time we can actually perceive electromagnetic energy is when it encounters interference of some kind. Lightening is an example of energy forces that can't be perceived until it meets interference in the atmosphere. However, even before the lightening erupts, the forces are there.

Electromagnetic fields are also present in and around the body whether or not we can see them with the naked eye or feel them. Electromagnetic forces in and around the body have been measured. And electrical currents of chick embryos have been seen to direct the positioning of the primitive streak. Unseen fields affect living systems, and living systems affect the unseen fields.

Health, or disease, can be seen as the result of influences of these unseen fields. Fields resonate with energy. The body resonates with energy. When the resonance of the living system and fields is synchronized, the system is healthy. When interference disrupts the synchronicity of the resonance, the system is diseased.

The most potent interference-generator of man is his thoughts. Positive thoughts feed and augment the positive energy of the fields. Negative thoughts cancel the positive, health enhancing energy of fields. Positive thoughts and attitudes restore the energy of fields depleted by negative-thinking.

The doctor's objective in helping patients is to help them replenish and revitalize their healing fields. This objective is met through a two-pronged procedure: 1) balancing the patient's internal energy to remove internal interference, and 2) projecting positive energy into the patient's field. B.E.S.T. Levels I and II procedures address the first objective. Level III procedures address the second. This book does not attempt to explain how traditional chiropractic works in removing interference, nor how Levels I and II are successful. This book was written to explain how thoughts (doctors' and patients') do affect healing.

Most doctors are quite comfortable with Levels I and II when they first encounter B.E.S.T. The rational for these procedures can be explained in terms with which most doctors are familiar and comfortable: muscle spindles, golgi tendon apparatus, righting reflex, sensory and motor systems. Level III, on the other hand, incorporates the practical, hands-on approach plus concepts that may be a little more difficult for scientifically-oriented doctors to accept graciously. However, when they see actual demonstrative evidence of patient improvement, they soon come to realize that there is more to chiropractic and healing than they were taught in school. And when they realize and understand that their attitude toward their patients, their technique, and themselves radically affects their success as healers, they accept and "own" the concepts.

Most doctors who expand their attitudes and practices to include B.E.S.T. Level III procedures find that their patients improve more and faster, they (the doctors) feel better and have more energy, and their practices grow as patients with a greater variety of chief complaints seek them out.

Level III exemplifies the concept that the more you give, the more you receive. As the doctor helps patients by contributing positive energy to the patients' energy fields, the doctor's own energy field is nourished. When the doctor projects positive energy into a patient's field, the patient starts resonating better with his field, feels better, and doesn't know what happened. And the best part of this is that the doctor doesn't even have to know the details of what caused the interference for the patient in the first place. In time, and with the doctor's help, the patient will learn to revise his own thinking to be more positive and keep himself healthy. Then the doctor's role is to keep the patient balanced through the stresses of life, and help the patient maintain positive healthful thoughts.

Positive energy is like sunshine. The sun always shines whether there are clouds between us and it or not. Clouds are interference that deflects the sun from our specific location. Positive energy is always available although sometimes, with prolonged interference, we tend to forget it's around. Negative thoughts produce interference. Unlike clouds, however, we can do something about negative thoughts.

The greatest gift a doctor can give a patient is the doctor's intent. Only by intending that healing or improvement occur will the doctor's efforts be rewarded the way he or she would like. Without intent, a doctor is a technician using only the conscious content of the cerebral cortex. Content decrees healing a science. Intent is the art of healing with feeling.

References

BOOKS

Bach, Marcus, Ph.D. *The Chiropractic Story.* Austell, GA: Si-Nel Publishing and Sales Co., 1968.

Beasley, Victor R., Ph.D. *Your Electro-Vibratory Body: A Study of the Life Force as Electro-vibratory Phenomena.* Boulder Creek, CA: University of the Trees Press, 1978.

Becker, Robert O., M.D., and Gary Selden. *The Body Electric: Electromagnetism and the Foundation of Life.* New York: William Morrow, 1985.

Becker, Robert O., M.D., *Cross Currents: The Promise of Electromedicine, The Perils of Electropullution.* Los Angeles: Jeremy P. Tarcher, Inc., 1990.

Black, Dean, Ph.D. *Health at the Crossroads: Exploring the Conflict Between Natural Healing and Conventional Medicine.* Springville, UT: Tapestry Press, 1988.

Burr, Harold Saxton. *Blueprint for Immortality: The Electric Patterns of Life.* Saffron Walden, GB: The C.W. Daniel Company Limited, 1972.

Carlson, Richard, Ph.D., and Benjamin Shield, ed. *Healers on Healing.* Los Angeles: Jeremy P. Tarcher, Inc., 1989.

Chopra, Deepak, M.D. *Quantum Healing: Exploring the Frontiers of Mind/Body Medicine.* New York: Bantam Books, 1989.

Chusid, Joseph G., M.D., and Joseph J. McDonald, M.D. *Correlative Neuroanatomy and Functional Neurology.* Los Altos, CA: Lange Medic al Publications, 1962.

Cousins, Norman. *Head First: the Biology of Hope.* New York: E.P. Dutton, 1989.

Davies, Paul, editor, *The New Physics.* Cambridge, UK: Cambridge University Press, 1989.

Dossey, Larry, M.D. *Space, Time & Medicine.* Boulder: Shambhala, 1982.

Dubos, Rene. *Mirage of Health: Utopias, Progress, and Biological Change.* New York: Harper & Row, 1959.

Encyclopaedia Britannica, Phillip W. Goetz, Ed in Chief. Chicago: Encyclopaedia Britannica, Inc., 1989.

Gerber, Richard, M.D. *Vibrational Medicine: New Choices for Healing Ourselves.* Santa Fe, NM: Bear & Company, 1988.

Guyton, Arthur C., M.D. *Textbook of Medical Physiology.* Philadelphia: W. B. Saunders Company, 1986.

Haldeman, Scott, D.C., Ph.D., M.D. *Modern Developments in the Principles and Practice of Chiropractic.* Norwalk, CN: Appleton-Century-Crofts, 1980.

Joy, W. Brugh, M.D., *Joy's Way: A Map for the Transformational Journey: An Introduction to the Potentials for Healing with Body Energies.* Los Angeles: J. P. Tarcher, Inc., 1979.

Justice, Blair, Ph.D. *Who Gets Sick: How Beliefs, Moods, and Thoughts Affect Your Health.* Los Angeles: Jeremy P. Tarcher, Inc., 1988 .

Krippner, Stanley and Daniel Rubin, ed. *The Kirlian Aura: Photographing the Galaxies of Life.* New York: Anchor Press, 1974.

Krystal, Phyllis. *Cutting the Ties That Bind: How to Achieve Liberation From False Security and Negative Conditioning.* Los Angeles: Aura Books, 1982.

Langman, Jan, M.D., Ph.D. *Medical Embryology: Human Development—Normal and Abnormal.* Baltimore: The Williams & Wilkins Company, 19 75.

Leonard, George. *The Silent Pulse: A Search for the Perfect Rhythm That Exists in Each of Us.* New York: E.P. Dutton, 1986.

Liebman, Michael, Ph.D. *Neuroanatomy Made Easy and Understandable,* Third Edition. Rockville, MD: Aspen Publishers, Inc., 1986.

REFERENCES

Litvak, Stuart, and A Wayne Senzee. *Toward a New Brain: Evolution and the Human Mind.* Englewood Cliffs, NJ: Prentice-Hall, Inc., 1986.

Magoun, H.I., Sr., *Osteopathy in the Cranial Field,* Third ed. Kirksville, MO: Journal Printing Co., 1976.

Morter, M.T., Jr., D.C. *Chiropractic Physiology: A Review of Scientific Principles as Related to the Chiropractic Adjustment with Emphasis on Bio Energetic Synchronization Technique.* Rogers, AR: B.E.S.T. Research Inc., 1988.

Morter, M.T., Jr., D.C. *Correlative Urinalysis: The Body Knows Best.* Rogers, AR: B.E.S.T. Research Inc., 1987.

Mountcastle, Vernon B., M.D., ed., *Medical Physiology,* Vol. II. St. Louis: C.V. Mosby Company, 1968.

Noback, Charles R., Ph.D., and Robert J. Demarest. *The Human Nervous System: Basic Principles of Neruobiology.* New York: McGraw-Hill Book Company, 1975.

Nordenstrom, Bjorn E.W., M.D. *Biologically Closed Electric Circuits: Clinical, Experimental and Theoretical Evidence for an Additional Circulatory System.* Stockholm, Sweden: Nordic Medical Publications, 1983.

Nuland, Sherwin B., M.D., *Doctors: The Biography of Medicine.* New York: Alfred A. Knopf, Inc., 1988.

Orten, James M., Ph.D., Otto W. Neuhaus, Ph.D. *Human Biochemistry,* Ninth edition. Saint Louis: The C. V. Mosby Company, 1975.

Oyle, Dr. Irving, *The Healing Mind: You Can Cure Yourself Without Drugs.* Millbrae, CA: Celestial Arts, 1975.

Pelletier, Kenneth R. *Mind as Healer, Mind as Slayer: A Holistic Approach to Preventing Stress Disorders.* New York: Dell Publishing Co., Inc., 1977.

Penrose, Roger (Rouse Ball Professor of Mathematics, University of Oxford), *The Emperor's New Mind: Concerning Computers, Minds, and The Laws of Physics.* (New York: Oxford University Press, 1989.

Restak, Richard M., M.D., *The Mind*. New York: Bantam Books, 1988.

Shafica, Karagulla, M.D., and Dora Van Gelder Kunz, *The Chakras and the Human Energy Fields*. Wheaton, IL: Theosophical Publishing House, 1989.

Shealy, C. Norman, M.D., Ph.D. and Caroline M. Myss, M.A. *The Creation of Health: Merging Traditional Medicine with Intuitive Diagnosis*. Walpole, NH: Stillpoint Publishing, 1988.

Sheldrake, Rupert. *A New Science of Life: The Hypothesis of Formative Causation*. Los Angeles: J.P. Tarcher, Inc., 1981.

Siegel, Bernie S., M.D. *Love, Medicine & Miracles: Lessons Learned About Self-Healing from a Surgeon's Experience with Exceptional Patients*. New York: Harper & Row, 1986.

Smith, Cyril W., and Simon Best, *Electromagnetic Man: Health and Hazard in the Electrical Environment*. New York: St. Martin's Press, 1989.

Srinivasan, T.M, Ph.D., ed., *Energy Medicine Around the World*. Phoenix, AZ: Gabriel Press, 1988.

Tompkins, Peter, and Christopher Bird. *The Secret Life of Plants*. New York: Avon Books, 1973.

Tuttle, W.W., Ph.D., Sc.D., and Byron A. Schottelius, Ph.D. *Textbook of Physiology*. St. Louis: The C. V. Mosby Company, 1961.

Watson, Lyall. *Beyond Supernature: A New Natural History of the Supernatural*. London: Hodder & Stoughton, 1986.

Westlake, Aubrey T. *The Pattern of Health: A search for a greater understanding of the life force in health and disease*. Berkeley: Shambhala, 1973.

REFERENCES

JOURNALS AND PERIODICALS

Barone, P., L. Narici, G.L. Romani, C. Salustri, V. Pizzella, and I. Modena. "Novel data analysis for synchronised spontaneous neuromagnetic activity," *Phys. Med. Biol.*, Vol 32, No. 1, 1987: 71-76.

Bassett, C.A.L. "Low energy pulsing electromagnetic fields modify biomedical processes," *Bioessays,* Vol. 6, No. 1, Jan 1987: 36-42.

Becker, Robert O., M.D., "Electromagnetism and the Revolution in Medicine," *Acupuncture & Electro-Therapeutics Res., Inst.,* J., Vol 12, pp. 75-79, 1987. A paper presented during the *2nd International Symposium on Acupuncture & Electro-Therapeutics,* held at the School of International Affairs, Columbia University, during October 16-19, 1986.

Benson, Herbert. "Your innate asset for combating stress," *Harvard Business Review,* Jul-Aug 1974: 49-60.

Chamberlain, David B., Ph.D., "The expanding boundaries of memory," For 4th Int. Congress on Pre & Perinatal Psychology, Amherst, Massachusetts, August 1989.

Cohen, David, Yoram Palti, B. Neil Cuffin, and Stephen J. Schmid. "Magnetic fields produced by steady currents in the body," *Proc. Natl. Acad. Sci.* USA, 77, 1980: 1447-1451.

Cope, Freeman W., "Discontinuous magnetic field effects (Barkhausen noise) in nucleic acids as evidence for room temperature organic superconduction," *Physiol. Chem. & Physics,* 10, 1978: 233-246.

Cope, Freeman W., "Magnetoelectric charge states of matter-energy. A second approximation, Part VII. Diffuse relativistic superconductive plasma. Measurable and non-measurable physical manifestations. Kirlian photography. Laser phenomena. Cosmic effects on chemical and biological systems," *Physiological Chemistry and Physics,* Vol 12, No. 4, 1980: 349-355.

Davenas, E., F. Beauvais, J. Amara, M. Oberbaum, B. Robinzon, A. Miadonna, A. Tedeschi, B. Pomeranz, P. Fortner, P. Belon, J. Sainte-Laudy, B. Poitevin & J. Benveniste, "Human basophil degranulation triggered by very dilute antiserum against IgE," *Nature*, Vol 333, June 30, 1988: 816-818.

Hall, Stephen S., "A Molecular Code Links Emotions, Mind and Health," *Smithsonian Magazine,* June 1989, pp. 62+.

Hamer, Ryke Geerd, from habilitation script presented at Tubingen University, October 1981.

Herman, Richard, M.D., James Mixon, Anne Fisher, Sc.D., Ruth Maulucci, Ph.D., and Joseph Stuyck, M.D., "Idiopathic scoliosis and the central nervous system: A motor control problem," *Spine,* Vol. 10, No. 1, 1985: 1-14.

Jaffe, Lionel F., and Claudio D. Stern. "Strong electrical currents leave the primitive streak of chick embryos," *Science*, Vol. 206, Nov 2, 1979: 569-571.

James, Russell. "Biomagnetics: A New Diagnostic Tool. *MI,* December 1980, p.74, 112-113.

Libet, Benjamin, "Neural Density: Does the Brain Have a Will of Its Own?" *The Sciences,* March/April 1989.

Marx, Jean L., "Electric Currents May Guide Development," *Science*, Vol 211, Mar 13, 1981: 1147-1149.

Miletich, David J., Akhtar Khan, Ronald F. Albrecht, and Anita Jozefiak. "Use of Heart Cell Cultures as a Tool for the Evaluation of Halothane Arrhythmia," *Toxicology and Applied Pharmacology* 70, 1983: 181-187.

Mueller, Larry. "A shock cure," *Outdoor Life,* June 1988: 64 ff.

Nakagawa, Kyoichi, M.D., (translation) "Magnetic field deficiency syndrome and magnetic treatment," *Japan Medical Journal,* No. 2745, Dec 4, 1976.

Nature, Vol. 333. June 1988.

Osteopathic Annals, 7:6, June 1979.

Papatheofanis, Frank J. "Review of the interaction of biological systems with magnetic fields," *Physiological Chemistry and Physics and Medical NMR*, 16, 1984: 251-255.

Patterson, Michael M., Ph.D., "Model mechanism for spinal segmental facilitation," *Journal of the American Osteopathic Association,* Vol 76, No. 1, Sep 1976: 62/121-72/131.

Raji, A.M. "Experimental study of the effects of pulsed electromagnetic field (Diapulse) on nerve repair," *J. Hand Surgery,* Vol. 9- B, No. 2, June 1984: 105-112.

Rivera, H., J.K. Pollock, and H.A. Pohl, "ac field patterns about living cells," *Cell Biophysics,* Vol 7, 1985: 43-55.

Stuchly, Maria A. "Human exposure to static and time-varying magnetic fields," *Health Physics,* Vol. 51, No. 2, (August) 1986: 215-225.

Thomsen, Dietrick, "Medicine's New Magnetic Field," *Science News,* Vol 123, June 1983: 408 ff.

Tourenne, Christian J., "A model of the electric field of the brain at EEG and microwave frequencies," *J. Theor. Biol.,* 116, 1985: 495-507.

Wisneski, Leonard A., M.D., "Biophychology: Overlapping Systems of Mind-Body-Environment," *Noetic Sciences Review,* June 26, 1989: 12 -16.

"When to believe the unbelievable," *Nature,* Vol 333, June 30, 1988: 787.

Index

acupuncture
   meridian 46
adrenal response 111
anesthesia 12
astro-osteoporosis 86
atom replacement 93, 94
attitudes 57, 112
Avogadro limit 65

Bacon, Francis 9, 18
bacteria 54
Becker, Robert O., M.D. 25
beliefs 115
biocycles 29
biodance 93
bioelectric pulses 106
Bio Energetic Synchronization
Technique (B.E.S.T.) 1, 2, 3, 23, 24, 59
   certification 29
   development 101, 133
   Levels I, II, III 135
biomagnetic fields 32
Biologically Closed Electric Circuits
(BCEC) 87, 88
Black, Dean, Ph.D. 53
body/mind 115
brain 51, 52, 59, 64, 66, 69, 123
   chemistry 90
   retina as part of 68
Burr, Harold S., 25

cell
   communication 56, 60
   electrical properties 51
   discovery 109
   division and differentiation 52
   information 2, 52, 59
   memory
   organizing principles
   tissue 53
   tumor 53
central nervous system 51, 64
chiropractic 17, 18, 29, 56, 59, 109
   advantage 126
cholates 44
cholesterol 44
communication 73
   among fields 26
   internal 59
content 123
cytoplasm 41

dc magnetic fields 33
deductive healing 13, 17, 132
defense physiology 57, 79, 111
Descartes, Rene 17

DNA 51, 53, 54, 61, 63, 93, 109, 115
double-blind studies 127

EEG 74, 89
effects 20, 133
   biological 92
EKG 74
electrical gradient 40
electricity 21
   currents 56
electromagnetic
   communication 50
   fields 24, 28, 31, 54, 57, 134
   forces 77, 87
   influence 89
   homeostasis 96
   oscillations 102
electron field 75-76
electronic matrix 90
electrons 39, 77, 81
electroweak force 35
embryo 49, 51, 52
   chick 50, 134
   developing 55, 57
emotion 57, 63, 65
energy
   fields 16, 75, 83
   information 78, 116
   positive 136
   negative 24, 52
   universal 99, 115
entrainment 103
environment
   external 19, 22
   internal 22
etheric body 54

field(s)
   around living systems 27, 54
   bioenergetic 54
   biomagentic 32
   electrodynamic 98
   environmental 26
   external 49, 57, 92
   geomagnetic 38, 92
   homeostasis 115
   influences 29, 39, 57
   internal 49, 57
   magnetic 26, 33, 92
   morphogenetic 63
   reflections 119, 121
frequency 81, 119

Galen 7, 8, 21
genes 93
genetic information 41

Gerber, Richard, M.D. 25, 77
gravity 21, 35

Hahnemann, Samuel, M.D. 18-19
Harvey, 5, 21
hippocampus 45
Hippocrates 7
holographic energy-field template 90
holography 3, 76
homeopathy 19
hope 124
hormones 50
Hunter, John 10
hypothalamus 45, 50, 66, 105

Imhotep 6
immune system 66
inductive medicine 13, 17, 132
infants 120-121
information 68, 116
   energy 55
   of cells 53
   of fields 77
   outside cell 52
Innate 17, 41
inspiration 68
intelligence, 54, 69
   universal 17
intent 123-129
   negative 125
   of doctor 3
   positive 125
interference 23, 79, 97

Josephson effect 45

Kirlian, 76
   photography 32, 90, 102
knowledge 79, 118
Kudu 73

Laennec, Rene 11 L-fields 90
life-field 89
lifestyle 19
Locke, John 9

magnetic fields 33, 37, 61, 85, 92
   deficiency 27
magnetic resonance imaging (MRI) 37
magnetic minds 89
magnetism 21, 84, 133
magnetometer 61
Maxwell, James Clerk 26
mechanistic approach 20
memory 61, 62, 70, 114
   suppressed 112
microwave 45
   foods 120

mind 15, 66, 110, 123
   influence of 16
Morgagni, Giovanni 10, 18

Nakagawa, Kyoichi, M.D. 27

Palmer, D.D. 17
Paraclesus, 8
Patagonians 118
"peas" 101
PEMF 89, 104, 105
perineural current 61
phantom leaf 64
photons 63
pineal gland 91
placebo 66, 70, 127-128
polarity 57
potential gradients 31, 106
pulsations 94-99, 101-107
   asynchronous 95
   bioelectric 106
   syncrhonized 96
pulsed electromagnetic
field (PEMF) 37

radio frequency 45
resonance 104, 119, 122, 124, 134
retina 68

self-disdain 113
self-esteem 113-114
sensory
   information 41
   system 41, 59
side effects 122
space 81
   information 41
   internal 40
SQUID 33, 34, 106, 109
stethoscope 11
stimulation
   electrical 56
subconscious 79
subluxations 23
superconduction 44
symptoms 23, 27, 85

tannin 62
thoughts 23, 66, 112, 116, 120
   negative 24, 57, 135
timing 23
toxicity 23

Vesalius, Andreas 9
Virchow, Rudolph 12

X-ray 45